NONI

Nature's Amazing Healer

NONI

Nature's Amazing Healer

NEIL SOLOMON, M.D., Ph.D.

New York Times Best-Selling Author
Former L.A. Times Syndication Health Columnist
Former CNN-TV Health Commentator
Maryland's first Secretary of Health and Mental Hygiene
Johns Hopkins Hospital Clinically Trained Physician

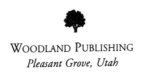

WOODLAND PUBLISHING
Pleasant Grove, Utah

This book is dedicated to my lovable and loved wife, Frema.

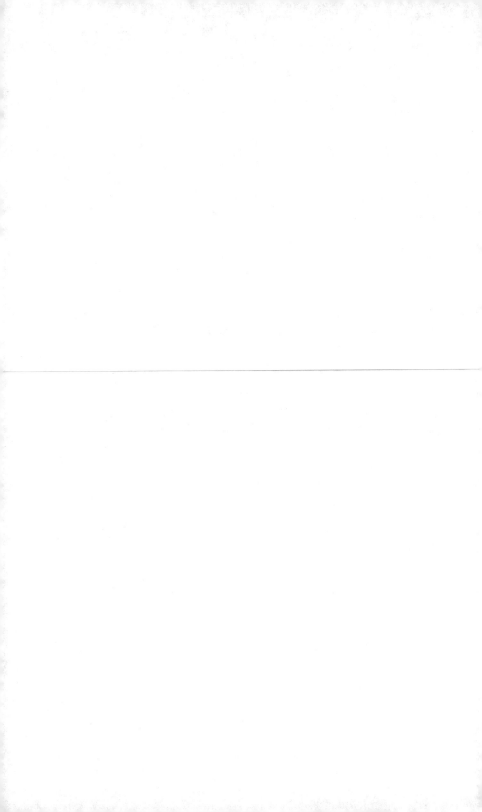

Contents

ACKNOWLEDGMENTS

I would like to acknowledge Dr. Ralph Heinicke, a scientist ahead of his time who brought us the "xeronine system" and its noni connection; I would also like to thank Dr. Anne Hirazumi, who helped delineate the noni–anticancer connection.

I also want to thank the following health-care professionals who so graciously shared their noni knowledge, information, and experiences with me:

Allan Bailey, B.Sc.Phm., naturopathic pharmacist, Canada
Bryant Bloss, M.D., Indiana
Richard T. Dicks, naturopathic educator, New Jersey
Frank Elaty, M.D., Florida
Scott Gerson, M.D., New York
Steven Hall, M.D., Washington
Mona Harrison, M.D., Washington
Dr. Delbert Hatton, California
Dr. Ralph Heinicke, Kentucky
Dr. Anne Hirazumi, Hawaii
Dr. Samual Kolodney, Pennsylvania
Dr. Jim Marcoux, Michigan
Dr. William T. Meier, Florida
Louise Morin, D.V.M., Pennsylvania
Dr. Alan Newman, Florida
Dr. Lois H. Rezler, California
Dr. Nelson T. Rivers , Indiana
Dr. Rick M. Smith, Florida
Dr. Stephen Schechter, California
Gary Tran, D.V.M., Kentucky

Preface

URING 1997 AND 1998 I researched the scientific evidence and field studies involving the island fruit noni to uncover its secrets as a medicinal agent. I logged hours and hours digging through case studies and reports from doctors and other experts, and thoroughly analyzed reports from an array of clinical trials. I also interviewed more than 40 doctors and other health professionals who had compiled data that collectively represented over 8,000 people who had used or were using noni.

As I was collecting these data, one of the questions I continually came back to was: "How can noni possibly help so many people with so many diverse health problems? What was its secret?" I concluded that, indeed, it does not help *everyone*—and it does not help with *all* health problems. However, 78 percent of the more than 8,000 noni users in our survey reported that it helped in some way, including fighting cancer, heart disease, digestive disorders, diabetes, autoimmune disorders, stroke, weight problems, and skin and hair problems.

This book will also take a closer look at the connection between bromelain, xeronine, proxeronine, and proxeroninase, four compounds that are emerging as the primary scientific reason behind noni's astonishing ability to aid the body in repairing the effects of a wide array of ailments and diseases.

The increased research into noni has yielded what Polynesian kahunas, or traditional healers, have known for ages: noni is a remarkable fruit and, layer by layer, scientists are steadily putting a stamp of approval on the plant and its medicinal abilities. Slowly but surely, noni is moving from the mystical world of tribal healers and island legends into the mainstream health arena, giving each of us the opportunity of benefiting from this powerful medicinal fruit.

Enjoy this book, and good health.

Neil Solomon, M.D., Ph.D.

1

Introduction: What is Noni?

MOST NORTH AMERICANS HAVE NEVER HEARD OF NONI, but that is sure to change. Noni, or *Morinda citrifolia,* which has long been hailed as a miracle plant in the primitive civilizations of ancient Polynesia, Asia, and Australia, is gaining more credibility as a genuine source of relief for many of the ailments and diseases that afflict modern-day societies.

Noni has been successfully used for over 2,000 years in Polynesia, China, India, and elsewhere in many different ways—as a dye, as food, and, most intriguingly, as an extraordinarily powerful medicine. It is the fruit's medicinal properties that have recently attracted a considerable amount of attention. Like aloe vera, kelp, papaya, pycnogenol and other botanicals, the extract of the noni plant has been demonstrated to improve a wide variety of health conditions.

In the latter half of the 1800s and throughout much of this century, these medicinal powers have largely been ignored; instead, the noni plant has been used primarily as a dye in clothing.

But a small, yet important movement of sorts has been taking place in the last few years of the twentieth century. Noni has taken its place at the forefront of alternative medicine because of its successful adjunctive treatment of ailments that vary from cancer to arthritis to high blood pressure and from weight control to skin and hair disorders.

Study after study, which we will address in this book, has yielded many positive results regarding the efficacy of noni in treating many of the most common ailments in modern times.

There is an old adage that is widely applied by the skeptic: "If it sounds too good to be true, it probably is." But there are always exceptions to this rule. So, what is noni, with its purported ability to combat dozens of health disorders? Is it the latest fad cure, or is it a legitimate source of relief—the balm of Gilead, as it were?

After talking to and studying the work of the world's leading noni researchers, after statistically evaluating the clinical responses of more than 8,000 people who took noni for a variety of health problems, and after reviewing feedback from over 40 physicians and health professionals and several traditional healers, the answer is clear: Noni is indeed a powerful medicinal fruit.

THE HISTORY OF NONI

The origins of noni are somewhat unclear, but because it is mainly found today in Tahiti and surrounding the ruins of ancient Polynesian villages on the islands of Hawaii, it is widely accepted that Polynesian settlers carried noni from their homeland to their new settlements in Hawaii about 1,500 years ago. These ancient Polynesian settlers probably brought along the noni plant for its varied uses. The bark yielded a red dye; the root, a yellow dye; the fruit served as a food in time of hunger. Most importantly, however, the leaves, fruit, and bark were also used as powerful medicines.

Polynesian legends are full of heroes and heroines who subsisted on the noni plant in days of hardship. In fact, one Tongan legend notes that the god Maui was restored to life by placing noni leaves all over his body.

While the historical accounts of noni are rare and somewhat mystical, the most fascinating aspect of the noni plant was the seemingly miraculous healing properties that natives all over the Pacific believed (and still believe) the noni plant possessed. In ancient times, all parts of the noni plant—the bark, leaf, fruit, root, flower, and seed—were valued for their efficacy on an impressive list of ailments. The noni plant was a principal method of treatment for nearly every disease imaginable, from reproductive system disorders to broken bones to infectious and inflammatory disorders to weight, skin and hair problems.

The noni plant can also be found in areas of Africa, Asia, Australia, and the Americas. In Central America, the noni has been known as a "pain killer" because of its abilities to relieve pain. In Burma, in the Malayan peninsula of Asia, the fruit was considered an edible food and was eaten raw or cooked. Other countries in the region ignored the culinary uses of noni and instead focused on its medicinal properties.

Generally, the noni plant has been similarly used throughout the world. It has long been used as a credible folk remedy for such ailments as fever, tuberculosis, hypertension, diabetes, malaria, liver ailments, and others. This widespread acceptance of noni as a medicinal remedy gives the plant an inherent credibility without even considering the modern scientific data that appears to justify its incredible healing properties and relatively few and minor side effects.

QUEEN OF THE GENUS

The genus *Morinda*, of the family *Rubiaceae*, is believed to include about 80 species of plants. According to H.B. Guppy, an English scientist who studied noni in the early 1900s, 60 percent of the 80 species of *Morinda* were confined to islands, large and small, in what is now Malaysia and in the Indian and Pacific oceans.

Today, only 20 of these species have been identified as having economic worth or being noteworthy in other ways. One species stands out as the "queen" of the *Morinda* genus for "its conspicuous features, its multiple uses, and its supreme ability to distribute itself on seacoasts far and wide without needing human aid."

This "queen," scientifically known as *Morinda citrifolia L.*, or noni, is a small, blossoming shrub with rounded branches and dark, glossy evergreen leaves that measure approximately a foot in length. Groupings of small, white flowers sprout at different times and eventually evolve into bumpy, egg-shaped fruit that are a few inches long and etched with many circular indentations or pits (many people think noni fruit resembles a small potato). The waxy yellowish-white skin of the fruit becomes thin and translucent when the fruit is ripe, and the tasteless, whitish pulp deteriorates into a very smelly (a "rotten cheese smell" is a common description of the odor of ripe noni), terrible-tasting semi-liquid that readily seeps through the skin of the fruit. The fruit contains numerous reddish-brown seeds that have bladder-like air sacs that give the seeds buoyancy in water. Although Guppy said the fruit quickly decayed when it fell into the ocean, he noted the seeds were extremely buoyant because each has a bladder-like cavity. In a remarkable study, he placed noni seeds in salt water that resembled ocean water, and after five weeks, found them "all afloat and sound." He concluded that noni seeds could float unharmed for many months. Because of Guppy's research, many noni experts have concluded that the ability of the noni seed to float in ocean water accounts for much of its great distribution.

The noni plant also merits recognition for its ability to flourish in even the harshest environments. It is very resistant to salt and salt water, and can resist the onslaught of drought for several months. Additionally, it isn't very finicky about soil, growing wild on the sandy shores of Australia, the rocky, volcanic shores of Hawaii, and even the limestone terrain of Guam. It appears that the best noni for medicinal purposes comes from pollution-free areas.

The fruit of the noni tree is edible, but its pungent taste and odor (TV star Robert Urich, who takes supplemental noni juice, recently told me it smells like his old baseball glove) have ensured that most people eat it only in times of famine. Early Hawaiians, for example, ate noni fruit only when there was nothing else to eat. Some groups are heavily dependent on the noni plant for food. In Samoa and Fiji, the raw or cooked fruit is a common complement to many meals. Australian natives are very fond of the fruit. In Burma, the unripe noni fruit is cooked in curries; the ripe fruits are eaten raw, usually heavily saturated with salt. The Burmese even roast and eat the seeds.

As evidenced, the applications of the noni plant are wide-ranging—everything from medicine to food to clothing dye. Its appellation as "queen" of the *Morinda* genus is quite appropriate.

NONI AS MEDICINE

In the context of this book, the most important characteristics of the noni fruit are its remarkable healing properties for a variety of ailments. Without getting into the scientific details of how noni acts as a healing agent (we'll examine that later), rest assured that a high percentage of people with assorted ailments who use or have used noni as part of their treatment reported astonishing success rates. The remainder of this book will examine the results of various research, including our survey of more than 8,000 noni users. We'll provide a more explicit explanation of the biochemical reactions that occur in the body when taking noni.

Remember that old saying we mentioned earlier? It goes something like this: "If it sounds too good to be true, it probably is." While this may be true in many cases, scientific data and stories from those who have taken noni point to its effectiveness. Although noni and its healing properties may sound too good to be true, in reality, noni may just be the medicinal miracle plant our deteriorating bodies have been craving in modern times.

2

How and Why
Noni Works

Keep in mind that the following is a light discussion of how noni interacts with the body to support a healing process. A more in-depth, scientific examination of how noni functions is included in later chapters of this book.

HOW DOES NONI WORK?

Dr. Ralph Heinicke, the world's premier researcher of noni, believes that noni helps in the normalization of abnormally functioning cells by delivering to the body the essential biochemical compound proxeronine, which cells then assemble into the alkaloid xeronine. Xeronine exhibits positive effects on cells, which results in most people feeling better. Understanding how the body makes xeronine (biosynthesis) is essential to understanding how noni works.

While at the Pineapple Research Institute in the 1950s, Dr. Heinicke isolated a crystalline material that belonged to none of the conventional biochemical compounds. Years later, he realized that this crystalline material was a critical component for the synthesis of the alkaloid xeronine. He also realized that the concentration of this material in the pineapple plant had decreased very significantly over the years because of soil micronutrient deficiencies. Today, by several orders of magnitude, noni fruit is the best source of this critical ingredient.

Dr. Heinicke believes that xeronine has an extremely important function in cells. First, xeronine incorporates itself into the structure of certain specific proteins; this change in the protein's structure allows it to concentrate the tremendous amount of energy contained in water to do various types of mechanical, chemical and electrical work in each cell. Obviously, these actions enable a normal cell to work more efficiently and help a damaged cell repair its deficiencies.

The most promising substance found in noni is proxeronine, which is converted by the body into xeronine, a critical biochemical compound involved in a wide range of normal human biochemical reactions. In inflamed areas, proxeronine leaks out of blood capillaries to enable the cells to produce free xeronine. Through a somewhat complex process, the free xeronine then reduces and prevents further inflammation in that area.

Mona Harrison, M.D., formerly assistant dean of Boston University School of Medicine, and chief medical officer D.C. General Hospital, reports that noni enhances the function of the thyroid and the thymus glands, which she believes act to fight off infections and other problems with the immune system. She even reports that noni helps to fight depression, possibly through its effect on brain hormones and neurotransmitters. Dr. Harrison further believes that frequency modulations in the body's energy may account for some of noni's positive actions. Noni juice has its own specific frequency; this frequency, along with xeronine and the other compounds in noni, is what adds to noni's therapeutic abilities. It stabilizes blood sugar, reduces menstrual cramping, and lessens the need for men with an enlarged prostate to urinate at night. In reviewing the literature, it appears that noni is a true adaptogen—it enhances the body's healing system regardless of the medical treatment a patient is receiving. As an adaptogen, noni brings the body into more normal balance; this state of being normal is called homeostasis. For example, if blood pressure is too high, noni helps lower it. If blood pressure is too low, noni helps raise it. If blood sugar is too high, noni helps lower it. If sugar is too low, noni helps raise it. Noni also acts in the same way if there is too much or too little acid in the body.

The fact that noni juice is teeming with compounds that have been scientifically proven to have a great deal of efficacy against myriad diseases is yet another indication that the tropical herb is a credible source of relief from many, many ailments.

So, is noni a cure-all? Does it cure cancer? Probably not. If that is true, is there any possible explanation that can be given for some of the positive observations that

Dr. Harrison recorded after her cancer patients took noni? There certainly is; however, we'll discuss it more in chapter 3.

I have spoken to descendants of ancient South Pacific healers who consider noni to be a sacred fruit. They aren't at all surprised by the incredible positive medical results that many people on the mainland experience with noni. Dr. Harrison concludes: "The modern world of medicine is finally starting to catch up to the knowledge of ancient times. We now have the instrumentation necessary to evaluate what it is about noni that allows it to cause such dramatic improvement in so many areas of the body. Noni, an ancient remedy, is finally being validated by breakthroughs in modern technology."

3

Indications for the Use of Noni Juice

A S MENTIONED PREVIOUSLY, NONI'S MEDICINAL APPLI-
cations are far-reaching and wide-ranging. It has
been shown to be effective against a list of diseases from A to Z, acne to zoonosis (an animal disease
like rabies or malaria that is communicable to man). This
chapter reports some of the findings from the doctors
and health experts interviewed for this book.

CANCER

Important research on the medicinal uses of noni was
presented at the 83rd, 84th, and 85th Annual Meeting of
the American Association for Cancer Research. A land-
mark paper from studies at the Departments of
Pathology and Pharmacology at the Johns Burns School
of Medicine in Honolulu, Hawaii was presented at the

83rd meeting in San Diego, California, in 1992. The findings were summarized in the Proceeding of the American Association for Cancer Research in an article titled "Anti-Tumor Activity of *Morinda citrifolia* on Intraperitoneally Implanted Lewis Lung Carcinoma in Mice." The mice fed noni fruit lived from 105 to 123 percent longer than mice that were not fed noni, and 40 percent lived for 50 days or more—a comparatively long time for mice suffering from cancer. The study was repeated numerous times, and each time the noni fruit was shown to significantly prolong the life of cancerous mice, in comparison to the cancerous mice that were not given the noni fruit. Simply put, these studies show that noni fruit may inhibit tumor growth. The increase in survival time averaged 119 percent after the administration of noni. There was an even greater increase in survival time when noni was administered with known anti-cancer medications such as adriamycin, 5-fluorourcil (5FU), or vincristine.

In support of the studies done in Hawaii, the journal *Cancer Letter* reported that Keio University and the Institute of Biomedical Sciences in Japan claimed isolation of a new compound from noni called damnacanthal. This work was done in the laboratory, not in humans. In layman's terms, what the damnacanthal in noni may do is encourage the genes in pre-cancerous cells to "believe" they are healthy cells, thereby preventing prolonged multiplication of the cells. In 1993, Tomonori Hiramatsu and three other Japanese researchers reported that after analyzing over 500 different plant extracts, the phytonutrient damnacanthal found in noni is "a new inhibitor of some precancerous cells."

HIGH BLOOD PRESSURE

In 1992, Dr. Isabelle Abbott, a recognized expert in botanical sciences, noted that the more common uses of noni include controlling diabetes, high blood pressure and cancer. I searched the literature to find which phytonutrients (foods with healing properties) in noni could help lower high blood pressure to normal levels. Scopoletin, a phytonutrient constituent of noni, dilates previously constricted blood vessels. This means that the heart does not have to overwork to pump against constricted (narrow) blood vessels. As a result, a normalization of the blood pressure takes place, which results in less wear and tear on the heart.

Scopoletin was first isolated from noni in 1993 by researchers at the University of Hawaii. It is believed that besides dilating blood vessels, scopoletin also binds to serotonin. Animal studies have shown that scopoletin can lower normal and high blood pressures to hypotensive levels, which are abnormally low blood pressure. However, in noni, scopoletin synergistically interacts with other nutraceuticals, which are foods acting as medicinals, to bring high blood pressure to normal, but not lower than normal. Noni has not been shown to bring normal blood pressure to hypotensive levels.

More recently, noni has been studied in the U.S. at Stanford University, the University of California at Los Angeles (UCLA), and the University of Hawaii; in England at the Union College of London; and in France at the University of Meets. Those studying it agree that in most cases noni can aid the lowering of high blood pressure.

I interviewed Scott Gerson, M.D., of the Mt. Sinai School of Medicine in New York, who completed a place-bo-controlled clinical trial to evaluate whether noni low-ered elevated blood pressure. For 14 weeks, Dr. Gerson studied nine patients—six males and three females. The high blood pressure patients were randomly selected and did not know that they were taking noni. They stayed on the same diet and did the same amount of exercise as before they started taking noni. Each patient acted as his/her own control. After taking noni, eight of the nine patients showed a decrease in blood pressure. On aver-age, their systolic (the top number of the blood pressure) decreased 7.5 percent, and their diastolic (the bottom number of the blood pressure) decreased 4 percent.

Dr. Gerson was the first to point out that although this was only a small clinical trial and not a super-scientific experiment, it nevertheless indicated that noni can lower high blood pressure. His findings were consistent with the results of our survey and other research. Of all the doctors I interviewed, not one told me that noni dropped elevated or normal blood pressure below nor-mal, and all reported that the side effects were almost nonexistent. Many noni users reported that their high blood pressure returned if they stopped taking noni, then returned toward normal upon reinstating a noni regimen.

Dr. Mona Harrison also reported that noni improves high blood pressure. One woman's blood pressure was 170/100 and her doctors could not lower it. After two months on noni, it dropped to a normal level of 130/80. She has continued to take noni and her blood pressure has remained normal for over 9 months. Dr. Samuel Kolodney of the Logan Square Family Clinic in Pennsylvania and Dr. Jim Marcoux of the Marcoux Clinic in Michigan both report that the majority of their hypertensive patients experienced a drop in high blood pressure levels toward normal levels after taking noni.

BACTERIAL INFECTION

In numerous studies, scientists and graduate students all over the world have corroborated noni's antibacterial properties.

In 1963, Oscar Levand, a graduate student at the University of Hawaii, reported that juice extract from the noni fruit showed remarkable abilities to ward off infection from several types of bacteria: *Salmonella typhosa*, several species of *Shigella*, *Pseudomonas aeruginosa*, *Proteus morganii*, *Staphylycoccus aureus*, *Bacillus subtilis* and *Escherichia coli* (commonly known as *E. coli*) are some of the major bacteria that were directly affected by noni. While many of these bacterial infections are unfamiliar to most people, rest assured that they all result in unpleasant sickness, grief, and even death. This does not suggest, however, that noni be used as a sole replacement for needed antibiotics.

PAIN

It has been accepted that one of noni's major benefits is its relief of most types of pain. From the Eastern medicine healers of Southeast Asia, to the Hawaiian kahunas (spiritual healers), to modern-day researchers like Dr.

Ralph Heinicke and clinical naturopaths like Dr. Steve Schechter, all parties agree that noni can and often does relieve pain.

But how noni works to relieve pain is not so easily agreed upon. Different theories have surfaced. Dr. Heinicke believes that pain relief is brought about by xeronine. Dr. Schechter, of the Natural Healing Institute of Naturopathy in California, believes that noni allows the body to heal itself (acting as an adaptogen), thus relieving pain. Who is right? I suspect they both are. And I suspect there are probably many other unknown substances in noni that contribute synergistically to pain relief.

Paul Alan Cox, one of the top ethnobotanists in the world, wrote in 1991 about how the dedicated kahunas passed noni pain treatment secrets down from generation to generation. My face-to-face conversations with Dr. Cox confirm what I have learned from personal communication with several kahunas. One of these kahunas, who was from Hawaii, said the magic of noni is "pule" (prayer). Another from a Maui temple said that the magic of noni has been handed down from generation to generation and that its healing power "comes from within."

Richard Dicks, a New Jersey naturopathic educator, cites his personal experience with noni. His son had severe bone disease and arthritis and experienced tremendous pain since he was very young. When Richard heard about noni from a friend, he decided to do his own detective work. For eight months he took noni himself and also gave it to his son without telling anyone.

Richard told me in an interview that noni was a "secret agent." His son's pain dissipated to the point that it was almost completely gone. He believes noni is effective because it helps cells quickly and effectively regenerate. Once this regeneration takes place, he believes people really start to reap the benefits. Richard summarizes by saying, "We're beginning to realize that we must get back to basics with our bodies. What it boils down to is either burn nutrients or burn your body. Noni saves our bodies by giving us the nutrients we need."

What does science have to say about noni's relief of pain? In 1992, Julia Morton, a botanist, reported that noni contains terpenes which are found in essential oils and have been shown to aid in cell synthesis and cell rejuvenation. It is also reported that xeronine has the ability to help normalize abnormal protein and subsequent cellular function, including brain function, where pain originates. Dr. Heinicke has accumulated data consistent with the explanation that xeronine and endorphins (feel-good hormones) occupy similar receptors. In 1990, Chafique Younos reported that Dr. Joseph Betz, a research chemist with the FDA's Division of Natural Products Center for Food Safety and Applied Nutrition, said that noni root is described "as having pain killing and tranquilizing properties."

In May of 1995, when I was an invited guest speaker at the 2nd International Pycnogenol Symposium in Biarritz, France, I had an opportunity to converse with some French scientists. It was there I learned that researchers at the Laboratory of Pharmacosny at the University of Meets in France had found that noni has a central analgesic effect. Simply put, the scientists told me that noni's effect on the brain is to relieve pain throughout the body. According to their studies, noni is 75 percent as effective as morphine sulfate in relieving pain. However, unlike morphine, noni is not addictive. Doctors and other health professionals interviewed believe that noni helped 87 percent of the more than 8,000 noni users in our survey who were suffering from varying degrees of pain.

INFLAMMATORY AILMENTS

We previously discussed how noni, which contains scopoletin, helped people control their high blood pressure. Noni also happens to be quite effective as an anti-inflammatory and as an antihistaminic agent. Medical literature has numerous reports of the successful treatment of arthritis, bursitis, carpal tunnel syndrome, and allergies with noni and the scopoletin compounds contained in the fruit.

This theory is well demonstrated by Bryant Bloss, M.D., faculty at the University of Louisville Hospital and orthopedic surgeon from Indiana. He describes his personal experience with noni and the experience of one of his patients:

> Before I used noni in my practice, I tried it myself and had a lot of personal success with it. I used to be unable to sleep on my stomach because of back pain. Noni not only took care of that, but it also relieved the pain in my left shoulder. Noni has also increased my energy level. My opponents on the ten-

nis court have noticed that my reaction time is much faster. Since then, I have used noni on about 70 of my patients. Fifteen of my patients with chronic back pain found that noni significantly relieved their pain. Eight other patients had knee pain from osteoarthritis, until noni made them almost pain-free. Several of my patients with Type II diabetes (adult onset, non-insulin dependent) lowered their blood sugar after taking noni.

One diabetic patient with chronic back pain found that for the first time in 15 years, he could bend over and pick up balls on the tennis court. He could also golf again without always being laid up afterward. The other day he told me that he has Bell's palsy (paralysis of part of the face). His family physician had told him that he'd be laid up for six weeks with a patch over his swollen eye. He doubled the amount of noni he was taking and in three days his symptoms were significantly improved.

Dr. Bloss' patients also use noni for other inflammatory ailments. Three asthma patients experienced much improvement in their asthmatic coughs after using noni. Many arthritic patients have experienced significant positive results. Two people, including a physician using noni, called to say that noni took away much of the stiffness in their hands within 24 hours.

Dr. Bloss reports that noni juice has been very effective as an anti-inflammatory for the majority of his patients. He offers it as a food supplement, not as a drug, and most of the patients choose to try it.

Most also continue to use it. In fact, our survey showed that 69 percent of the people who took noni continued to use it and refused to give it up. Dr. Bloss sums up noni in this fashion: "Noni has improved not only my own life, but the lives of many of my patients." The same sentiment was expressed by two graduates of Logan College of Chiropractics, Dr. George Squires of Indiana, and Dr. William Meier of Florida.

VETERINARY MEDICINE

Island folklore suggests that it was common for pigs to eat noni in the wild. It is also says that those pigs who ate noni were healthier and had more stamina than animals that did not. Dr. Gary Tran, a veterinarian graduate from Oklahoma State University and staff at the Animal Emergency Center in Kentucky, who has treated over 2,000 animals with noni, reports that animals as well as humans respond positively to noni. In his veterinary practice he incorporates both traditional and holistic medicine and has used noni in his treatments.

Dr. Tran first heard about noni two years ago, and was skeptical of its effectiveness. Finally, he convinced himself to try it. The day he made the decision to try noni as a dietary supplement, his aunt called and told him that her daughter was dying of AIDS. Dr. Tran sent noni to his aunt that very day. He reports that noni helped his cousin so much that he decided to give it to his immediate family. It helped his wife's chronic fatigue syndrome and depression, as well as his son's debilitating migraine headaches. (Our survey of more than 8,000 noni users showed that after taking noni, 87 percent had headache relief, and 77 percent were helped with depression). It even eased his own arthritis pain and asthma.

The results were so dramatic for his entire family that he decided to use it on the four-legged patients at his clinic. Dr. Tran reported that more than 90 percent of the animals have responded very positively. He notes that "noni is not only wonderful for alleviating pain, it's also antihistaminic, anthelmintic (rids animals of worms), anti-inflammatory, analgesic, and anti-carcinogenic." He believes that it strengthens the immune system's ability to fight viral infections. He further believes that noni heals and rejuvenates sick tissue, controls vomiting, counteracts poisons, and stabilizes animals that are in shock. And it takes care of the inflammation associated with joint problems, arthritis, sprains, and fractures. Noni also helps organs to heal more quickly, reverses some neurological disorders, helps spinal cord injuries, and enables animals to recover from comas more quickly. Dr. Tran no longer needs to use painkillers, muscle relaxants, or steroids on most of his animal clients; instead, he uses noni juice.

Dr. Tran also reports some dramatic cases of animals being helped by noni. One owner accidentally ran over his dog because it was sleeping under the car, leaving the dog hobbled with several severe fractures. Dr. Tran set the broken bones in a cast and gave the dog a daily dosage of noni. In two weeks, the animal had completely healed. He believes the healing took place much faster because he used noni juice.

Another dog had been hit by a car and was suffering from severe internal injuries. Dr. Tran could not surgically repair the dog's internal injuries because of their severity. Instead, he started the dog on a regimen of intravenous fluids and noni juice by mouth. The dog's condition stabilized very quickly; consequently, Dr. Tran decided to operate. When he cut the dog open, he was astounded when he saw that many of the dog's most important internal organs had been ruptured, but were now under repair. The dog surely should have been dead. Dr. Tran believes that noni helped to save the dog, which eventually made a complete recovery.

Dr. Tran notes: "I have found that noni is the most wonderful substance which a doctor can use in this line of work. In all my 35 years of practicing traditional and holistic veterinary medicine, I haven't seen any other product that is as versatile as noni. If I were banished to a remote island and could bring only one health product, it would definitely be noni."

I interviewed another veterinarian, Dr. Louise Morin, a graduate of University of Pennsylvania Veterinarian Medicine, and currently practicing with her husband at the Delaware Valley Animal Hospital, who bridges the gap between traditional and holistic animal health. She, too, agreed that noni juice helps many of the animals she treats, stating that it is especially effective for pets with arthritic problems, and is virtually without side effects.

4

The Effectiveness of Noni Juice

LET'S GET AWAY FROM THE SCIENTIFIC DISCUSSION FOR the time being and focus on the stories involved with noni. We'll continue the discussion of noni's astonishing medicinal properties by discussing the first doctor I interviewed: Mona Harrison, M.D., a knowledgeable physician from Washington.

To better help her patients, Dr. Harrison studies the latest alternative food supplements on the market to determine what effects—good or bad—they may have on her patients. She first learned about noni in 1997 from one of her staff members who, after only two weeks of taking the juice, had noticed dramatic improvement of her varicose veins and the near-vanishing of a chronic digestive ailment that had troubled her for years.

Intrigued by the positive results, Dr. Harrison sent a package containing noni to several of her patients around the country, advising them to try the food supplement.

The results were spectacular. One woman was suffering from kidney cancer with metastases (the malignant cells had migrated to her lung and brain), and her oncologist had given her only two weeks to live. She immediately began taking Dr. Harrison's noni and, according to her stunned oncologist, her lung X-rays cleared. The patient continued taking noni and the quality of her life vastly improved.

Another of Dr. Harrison's patients, who had developed liver cancer, became subject to sporadic bouts of swelling from excessive fluid in her abdominal area. After seven days of supplementing her diet with noni, the abdominal swelling had significantly decreased. When her oncologist examined her abdominal fluid, it was free of cancer cells.

Doctors like Dr. Harrison and other health professionals who were interviewed for this book believe that noni sparked at least minor to moderate improvement in 67 percent of their cancer patients.

Arthritis is another condition that may respond to noni. One of Dr. Harrison's patients who reported positive results was a woman who had suffered from degenerative arthritis for 20 years. Her knees had been replaced, but it did little to alleviate the pain. She still had to walk with a cane and had a difficult time getting up from a sitting position. After using Dr. Harrison's noni for just 72 hours, she was able to get up from a soft-cushioned sofa and move most of the way across the room without a cane—or pain. This was a dramatically positive experience for the patient. She knew that noni helped because it was the only variable that had changed in her life.

Doctors like Dr. Harrison and other health professionals who were interviewed for this book believe that noni has helped 80 percent of their arthritic patients.

A woman with macular degeneration, seen as a dark spot on the back of her eye, also received the noni package from Dr. Harrison. The woman's vision had deteriorated so much that she was essentially blind. Worse yet, she had little hope of her vision ever improving. She had been to some of the premier ophthalmologists at the top medical centers in the country, but they had been stymied by her ailment and had been unable to help her. After two and a half weeks of taking noni, her sight had markedly improved and some regeneration had taken place.

According to Steven Hall, M.D., of Providence Hospital in Washington, another physician I interviewed who uses noni, "not only does noni provide many benefits on its own, but it also increases the effectiveness of other treatments." He reports success in treating patients with "inflammation problems such as arthritis, tendonitis, bursitis, or carpal tunnel [syndrome]." He has found that "noni is incredible because it offers help to people who could not be helped by traditional medical science." His results are consistent with the previously reported positive response from 78 percent of noni users.

To see if these positive results obtained by physicians using noni were consistent with the results obtained by naturopathic clinicians, I interviewed Dr. Schechter and other naturopaths, Richard Dicks and Alan Bailey, M.H. These naturopathic educators are huge supporters of noni and, along with Dr. Schechter, have treated hundreds of patients with the tropical fruit. They are very impressed with the variety of illnesses that respond to noni. But, by the nature of their naturopathic practices, they have few clients who are only taking noni and no other supplement and/or medication. The great majority of these people take other natural supplement remedies as part of their naturopathic treatment regimen. But when they add noni to their treatment program, there is usually additional improvement.

Most of the doctors and other health professionals I interviewed supported Dr. Schechter's observations. The beneficial effects of noni are further substantiated by many of their patients and/or clients. During my interviews, I was able to find 93 people who for a period of time took only noni and no other food supplement or medications. Table 1 shows the results.

Allan Bailey, a naturopathic pharmacist and master herbalist from Canada, reports that he first heard of noni during a visit to French Polynesia. The Polynesian healers referred to noni as one of the most important plants they had used in their herbal therapies. One researcher in French Polynesia who had studied the uses of more than 300 herbs felt that noni was one of the most vital, if not the most vital, healing plants available. Alan took some noni home and began to take it regularly. It helped him to attain more restful sleep. As a result, he felt more energized and refreshed when he woke. He noticed that he

Condition	# who took only noni	# helped by noni*
Cancer, lessened symptoms	9	5
Heart disease, decreased symptoms	13	8
Stroke	5	3
Diabetes, type 2	6	4
Energy, increased	18	14
Sex, enhanced enjoyment	5	4
Obesity, lost excess weight	24	15
Fuzzy thinking, helped clear	11	6
Smoking, stopped	24	13
Arthritis, lessened symptoms	42	29
Pain, including headaches, decreased	43	31
Depression, lessened symptoms	14	9
Allergy, decreased symptoms	8	5
Fibromyalgia, decreased symptoms	11	6
Digestion, improved	15	10
Breathing, improved	27	17
Cholesterol, lowered	16	14
Cluster headaches, reduced	19	10
Longer/stronger fingernails	5	3

* 74 out of the 93 people who took only noni had 2 or more problems existing simultaneously that were helped by noni. Over half the people were clinically helped with one or more of their problems after taking nothing but noni.

Table 1: Results of sole noni supplementation

could do more during the day than he had in the past because noni gave him added energy and endurance.

Due to his success with noni, Alan decided to give noni to his diabetic mother. She had tiny sores all over her arms and legs that had not responded to any treatment for over three years. He had her take noni three times a day. After six weeks, he reported that the sores cleared. Noni also gave his mother more energy and more enthusiasm to exercise, which helped control her elevated blood sugar. Doctors and other health professionals interviewed believe that noni helps 83 percent of their diabetic patients.

Alan also has a close friend whose arms had been wasting away and who had violent arm and leg twitches. After two weeks of taking noni, he called Alan to tell him that, "On the seventh day of taking noni, I didn't have any leg twitches, and I started to feel more strength in my arms." That was six months ago and he's continuing to improve. Noni has done so much good for Alan's family that he now recommends it to most of his clients.

Another benefit of noni was illustrated in the treatment of one of Alan's patients. This man had an ulceration on his leg that was prone to erupting, and the skin around the ulcer was itchy and irritated. After he ingested noni and applied it topically for a few weeks, he reported that the ulcer was completely healed and the surrounding area didn't bother him anymore. Now, the circulation and color are coming back. He still soaks a bandage in noni and wears it on the spot where the ulcer was to make sure noni is always working on the area. He doesn't want the problem to return.

Alan reports that noni has generated more calls from his clients because of its benefits than any other food supplement he has ever recommended. From the experiences that people have shared, he feels that noni has universal applications and should be included as a part of everybody's daily nutrition. He believes that it helps us to absorb essential nutrients from our diets and supplements—in essence, noni is the missing piece of the health puzzle. Dr. Nelson Rivers, a holistic pharmacist from Indiana, has spoken to many noni users and is convinced that noni has a unique role in helping us stay healthy.

Dr. Delbert Hatton, a chiropractic physician from Sports Clinic in California, also cites his personal experience with noni's therapeutic properties. For about forty years, he had a constant nagging ache in his lower back from unevenly formed vertebrae. The pain prevented him from doing even normal household activities. After only six weeks of taking noni, the pain disappeared. He began recommending noni to his patients last fall. Since then he has had nothing but success with it.

The most amazing situation Dr. Hatton cites concerns a woman with AIDS. Since she has been taking noni, her T-cell count (a measure of resistance to the AIDS virus) has gone from 169 to 400, and her symptoms have stabilized!

Dr. Hatton also has a relative with lung cancer whose tumors have decreased in size since he has been taking noni. In support of Dr. Hatton, Dr. Ralph Heinicke (a pioneer in the field of noni research) reported to me that he knew of several cancer patients whose cancerous lesions decreased while on noni. He believes that while noni does not cure cancer, it allows the person's cancerous cells to function more normally. He believes that while cancer cells, after exposure to noni, continue to divide, they do so over a shorter period of time.

Another use of noni was evidenced several years ago when a patient of Dr. Hatton was traumatically injured in an auto accident. He broke several ribs, his shoulder, and his knee. Since then, he has had a lot of problems with arthritis resulting from the accident, especially in his knee. Days after he started using noni juice, the pain in his knee went away and he had a gradual decrease in the pain in his ribs and shoulder. Now, he is relatively pain-free.

Another of Dr. Hatton's patients broke the bones in her ankle and had lingering pain and swelling in the injured area for a year and a half. Ten days after she started taking noni, the pain and swelling decreased. Dr. Hatton attributes this to noni's ability to open up the cell wall, allowing nutrients to be absorbed and waste material to dissipate from the diseased or damaged cells. Dr. Hatton concludes: "I would recommend noni to anyone with any kind of health problem."

The kind of results reported by Dr. Hatton were very similar to the results reported by the kahunas (or healers) of the islands of the Pacific. They used noni "to treat health problems ranging from thrush to rheumatism. Intestinal worms, fevers, and skin infections were among the most common ailments treated by this French Polynesian cure-all."

Alexander Dittmar, an herbologist, published a comprehensive list of all the known uses of noni by the kahunas. I modified the list after traveling to Hawaii and speaking with some modern-day kahunas who referred me to some very sophisticated clinical practitioners. They told me how noni helps normalize the function of pre-cancerous tissue, enhances macrophage and lymphocyte activity, regulates the thymus, and helps with arthritis.

They even told me that noni helps relieve stress. This is reminiscent of what Dr. Scott Gerson told me. He said that noni helped him, especially with time-pressure— that is, the stress caused when he has to complete a task by a certain deadline. He feels that noni helps him react to that stress in a constructive way. Our survey of more

Abscess	Alcoholism
Allergies	Appetite, loss of
Arthritis	Asthma
Chest, burning in	Childbirth, tonic for
Chronic fatigue syndrome	Cigarette smoking
Cough, sore throat	Depression
Digestive cleanser	Drug abuse
Drug addiction	Eczema
Fever with vomiting	Gum disease, sore
Gums, inflamed or sore	Heart disease
High blood pressure	Indigestion
Infection of mouth and gums	Kidney/bladder problems
Lung problems	Menstrual problems
Obesity	Pain, generalized
Precancerous condition	Psoriasis
Skin, spreading of dark spots	Stress
Swelling, abdominal/ankle	Urinary tract ailments
Wounds, fractures and boils	

Table 2: Conditions reported by kahunas and island doctors to have responded to noni

than 8,000 noni users shows that 71 percent can better handle stress after taking noni.

After exhaustive interviewing of the nonmedical Hawaiian kahunas, the closest I could come to having them name a quantitative number of people who had benefited from noni was "most people."

Fortunately, I was able to compile Table 3 from a statistical analysis of the data I obtained from a survey of more than 40 doctors and other health-care professionals who have taken noni and/or given it to over 8,000 people. Seventy-eight percent reported being helped for one or more of their health problems after taking noni.

Dr. Schechter states, "As a clinical therapist, I have seen noni generate significant, even profound, therapeutic benefits for both prevention and self-help of a wide range of health problems." Table 4 lists some scientifically documented benefits of noni reported by Dr. Schechter, who saw the clinical benefits of noni on his

Conditions Reported to respond to noni	# Who took noni for that condition	% Helped*
Cancer, lessened symptoms	847	67%
Heart disease, decreased symptoms	1,058	80%
Stroke	983	58%
Diabetes, Types 1 and 2	2,434	83%
Energy, increased	7,931	91%
Sexuality, enhanced enjoyment	1,545	88%
Muscle, increased body-building	709	71%
Obesity, lost excess weight	2,638	72%
High blood pressure, decreased	721	87%
Smoking, stopped	447	58%
Arthritis, lessed symptoms	673	80%
Pain, including headaches, decreased	3,785	87%
Depression, lessened symptoms	781	77%
Allergy, decreased symptoms	851	85%
Digestion, improved	1,509	89%
Breathing, improved	2,727	78%
Sleep, improved	1148	72%
Fuzzy thinking, helped clear	301	89%
Well-being, increased feeling of	3,716	79%
Mental acuity, increased alertness	2,538	73%
Kidney health, improved	2,127	66%
Stress, helped cope with	3,273	71%

* Pooled percentage of people who experienced objective and/or subjective improvement of their signs and/or symptoms after taking noni. *The majority of noni users who did not get optimal results failed to do so because they took a lesser dose and/or took it for a shorter time than what was recommended, or simply responded for unknowable reasons.*
   ** Noni can be taken together with all other medications—there are virtually no negative interactions. In some situations, noni can allow other medications to act more efficiently. You should tell your health professional that you are taking noni as your physician might want to decrease the dose of the medication prescribed.
   *** Side effects were minimal. Less than 5 percent had loose bowel movements, a slight belch or developed a mild rash. The belch and loose bowel movements disappeared when the dose was decreased. The rash cleared within 72 hours after the person stopped taking noni.
   **** Noni was reported to be safe for pregnant and/or nursing mothers.

Table 3: Conditions Helped by People Who Took Noni (n=>8,000)

patients. There are many more claims of benefits, but, as yet, no confirming research.

After reviewing medical literature and speaking with health professionals who recommended noni to over 8,000 people, as well as talking with many of those who

Abdominal pains	Abdominal swelling
Abscesses	Anticancer activity
Antibiotic and Antimicrobial	Arthritis
Backache	Balanced nutrition
Burns	Chest infections
Dark spots on skin	Deficient Macrophages/Lymphocytes
Depression	Diabetes (Type 2)
Diaphragmatic hernia	Diarrhea
Dry or cracked skin	Eye complaints
Heart disease	High blood pressure
Infection of mouth/gums	Inflamed, sore gums
Inhibits early chronic fatigue syndrome	Intestinal worms
Regulates thymus	"Sick People Syndrome"
Sore throat with cough	Stroke
Tonic after childbirth	Toothaches
Tuberculosis	Urinary tract ailments
Virus problems	Wounds, fractures and boils

Table 4: Some Scientifically Documented Benefits of Noni

took noni and shared their experiences with me, I concluded the following:

- Noni helps many people (78 percent) for many but not all conditions.
- Noni exerts positive effects quickly in many people, and most people experience results within days to weeks. However, you should commit to taking noni for six months before deciding how much it helps.
- Noni is essentially nontoxic, and side effects, if any, are minimal and are totally reversible.
- Noni works synergistically with other food supplements and/or medications.
- Noni probably helps prevent the development of various disorders, and works optimally in conjunction with other antioxidants.
- Noni is reported to be safe for children and for pregnant and lactating mothers.

5

Some Case Studies

DR. STEVE SCHECHTER, DIRECTOR OF THE NATURAL Healing Institute in Encinitas, California, is one of the most enthusiastic and public supporters of noni. He pointed out in our interview for this book that there has been a wealth of information supporting the traditional uses and health benefits of noni.

According to Dr. Schechter, noni has long been used safely and effectively for chronic pain; in fact, he believes that noni's greatest value may be in alleviating pain. Two of the plant's traditional names are "pain-killer tree" (in the Caribbean islands) and "headache tree" (in Asia).

Dr. Schechter has used noni to treat numerous clients who were suffering from chronic pain due to different reasons. He told me of the many case studies from people across the United States who have successfully used noni to rid themselves of debilitating pain.

With all of this positive information regarding noni and its ability to relieve pain, the question arises: Can noni relieve pain without having toxic side effects? According to the feedback from Dr. Schechter's clients and others, the answer is an apparent "Yes".

In 1990, researchers found that "the administration of noni extract shows a significant, dose-related, central analgesic activity in mice." An analgesic is a substance that reduces or eliminates pain. The researchers went on to say that the "noni extract did not exhibit any toxic effects."

Dr. Schechter supports these findings with reports that chronic severe pain such as regular debilitating headaches, neuromuscular pain, and joint pain can be relieved with noni—and sometimes, results happen surprisingly fast.

Following are some of Dr. Schechter's case studies that examine specific ailments and disorders for which noni can be used.

MIGRAINES AND CLUSTER HEADACHES

Tom, an active, athletic patient who suffered from two or more migraines a week (along with a chronic shoulder condition that had caused him pain for years), was taking an acetaminophen-based pain killer with little success. The pharmaceuticals were disrupting his liver function, as evidenced by blood tests that showed liver damage. Dr. Schechter suggested to Tom that he try taking noni. After two weeks, Tom reported that he had no more migraines or shoulder pain. For the last seven months, he has been pain free.

Pam, a secretary working in a high-pressure office, had right-sided cluster headaches, neck pain, and dizziness. Again, Dr. Schechter suggested noni. After nine days, the headaches and pain were eliminated. After 18 days, there was no more dizziness and Pam also reported having more energy. Her husband, shocked by the results, decided to try noni for himself. They both reported more vitality, including greater sexual energy, which, Dr. Schechter believes, is a direct result of greater internal health. Pam and her husband's increased sexual vitality correlates with the information gathered from the more than 8,000 noni users studied for this book. In fact, 88 percent of them noticed improvement in their sexual performance.

I believe that Pam and her husband's increased energy was a direct result of an altered energy syndrome (AES), a condition I noted while serving on the Osler Medical Service at the Johns Hopkins hospital in 1961. I saw several patients at the hospital who were definitely ill—but their laboratory tests were normal or just slightly off of normal. These patients had previously been called "crocks" by some health professionals—but I still maintain, over 35 years later, that many of these "crocks" had legitimate medical problems. The problem was that in those days, we did not have sophisticated enough tests to diagnose many abnormal conditions. Many of those patients were referred to psychiatrists, when they should have been referred for energy testing. When I tested their energy levels, I found many had an altered energy state. To describe these people, I coined the term "altered energy syndrome." Pam and her husband were probably suffering from a similar condition. Like Pam and her husband, these patients probably would have benefited from food supplements such as noni, antioxidants, pycnogenol, shark liver oil, aloe vera, selenium, herbs, algae, chromium, beta carotene, vitamins A, C, E, zinc, glutathione, folic acid, vitamin B12, lipoic acid, bioflavonoids, proanthocyanidins (PACs) and others. It is now suspected that noni may help harness the energy released from the body's binding and release of hydrogen. This allows the body more "firepower" for cells to function more normally and for damaged cells to repair themselves more quickly.

CHRONIC PAIN

Gary, a dedicated athlete, learned of noni from Dr. Schechter. Gary says, "I was a two time All-American at Cal State Haywood in the triple jump. Currently, I act as the Sports Director of Team Fitness. I am still actively competing in track and field. I was having pain in my left knee and was not able to give my maximum effort during my training routine. I started taking noni, and after a few days, I noticed a distinct difference. I was no longer experiencing the pain, and I was able to perform at a higher level from an increase in energy. Noni has given me the ability to train at 110 percent without pain and has reduced my recovery time significantly."

Tim used noni for a different kind of pain. He says, "In 1992 I developed a crippling, painful condition— like shin splints—in my feet. I had gone to podiatrists and had custom inserts made for my shoes, tried different medications and never really had any quantifiable results with any of those types of treatment. A good friend introduced me to noni. When I started taking noni I wanted to believe, but I wasn't sure if it was really having any effect. But about two weeks into taking noni, I had total relief from the pain that had been plaguing me for the past six years.

"What I'm really excited about is another condition I have been fighting in my left hip. I don't know what it is. I have been to chiropractors, other doctors, and tried medications. It is a crippling type pain that is so irritating. I doubled my dosage and after a couple of days I noticed a dulling of the pain; currently, I have absolutely no pain. Regardless of the doctors' inability to diagnose the problem, the important issue is the result I have gotten from noni. To me it came down to a "quality-of-life" issue. Battling the pain has been continually aggravating and draining; it has affected my relationships with others and ultimately had a detrimental effect on my life. Now, noni has helped me overcome these things."

Blaine, from Washington state, says, "I am a professional basketball player in Puerto Rico, and I have been having some severe back pain for quite a while. Playing basketball can be very physical and, with all of the positioning as well as jumping, can be very hard on the back and uncomfortable." Along with the physical stress of playing a demanding sport, Blaine was also in a car accident and received a great deal of damage in his lower back. He explains, "The pain in my back has been unbearable. But I started taking noni and I noticed the pain and swelling around my lower back have completely gone away. Noni has also increased my strength and stamina greatly."

Earl, of New York City, tells quite an amazing story about the benefits of noni. He says, "As an officer for the Department of Corrections, I found myself in a major prison fight in the winter of 1985. I was pinned underneath a 1,000 pound vending machine and, as a result, my left shoulder was pushed 7 inches downward into my chest. During the last nine years, I've had four major surgeries and have not been able to lift my arms above my head or been able to sleep for more than 15 minutes at a time on either side. Even the most powerful prescription drugs did not ease my pain. But after taking noni for two weeks, I now sleep all night and can lift my arms above my head. I thank my wife, Amy, for always being there for me during those rough years, and I thank noni, which has made a huge difference in every moment of my daily life."

As noni helps relieve the pain associated with various problems and disorders, it does contribute to a more restful sleep. In fact, in the survey of over 8,000 noni users, 72 percent reported improvement with their sleep.

Ken, of Albuquerque, New Mexico, says, "I have farmed all my life, but about six years ago my brother accidentally ran into me with his four wheel all-terrain vehicle. This damaged a disc in my lower back, which pinched the sciatic nerve and sent sharp pains down my left leg every time I moved around. About three weeks ago a friend, Jason, called me and told me I should try a new product made from some fruit. I was very skeptical at first. But after Jason explained to me about noni, I became very excited. I've tried every pain reliever seen on TV—aspirin, Tylenol, Advil—all without any real results. I even started visiting the local chiropractor every week and although it helped, I still had pain. I asked my doctor about it and he told me (and I quote), 'Well, Ken, you'll just have to learn to live with the pain.' That was sure exciting news! If you've ever had back pain as bad as mine you'll try about anything short of surgery, especially if you have to go out and load 20 tons of wheat or baled hay onto a truck. But now, after only five days of using noni, my pain is 99 percent gone. I feel so good I went outside and started working in my garden, doing lots of bending, lifting, and standing—all with no more pain in my back. I feel better than I have in years."

Louis, of New Orleans, says, "I am 62 years of age and I used to have a hard time getting up in the morning and going to the bathroom. I was holding on to the walls, bed, and furniture until I got there and five or ten minutes later I could barely drag myself out. Then, two weeks ago I was introduced to noni, and within one day I noticed a difference. The pain was no longer there, so I continued taking noni. To this day I have no pain whatsoever. I have even had the energy and the will to go out and walk one and a half miles a day for the last two weeks. I feel wonderful, and this morning I got on the scale and am down almost 5 pounds. The only thing I did differently to lose weight was take noni. It is great and I recommend it to everyone."

Losing weight can be one of the excellent benefits of noni. The survey of over 8,000 noni users showed that after taking noni, 72 percent reported that they lost weight.

IMPROVED PHYSICAL ACTIVITY

Another of Dr. Schechter's patients is Clint, marketing director for a fitness club in Dallas, Texas. He says, "Taking noni has clearly been a positive experience. I run 3 miles three times a week and I've had some pain in my left knee. As a result of taking noni, I feel no pain. Noni has allowed me to run longer and faster. I feel stronger and really good from this. All you have to do is try it and experience the difference."

I told Clint's story to a friend of mine, Hal Katz, chairman of a very successful conglomerate of insurance corporations in Maryland. He is a decidedly youthful-looking 51 years old, probably as a result of his extensive knowledge of the latest antiaging food supplements and those that are ideal for developing muscle mass. He is very tuned in to his body, and listens when his body talks. He started taking noni, and after three days felt that he definitely had more energy. After six weeks he believed that he had increased muscle mass. He now works out more intensively than he did before. When he started taking noni, he had been taking pycnogenol and shark liver oil (both of which he continues to take). His friends say he never looked better.

Just as these people improved their physical appearance with noni, 71 percent of the more than 8,000 noni users surveyed said they looked like they had larger muscles. It might have been because they had more energy and thus exercised more. Hal also told me of an unexpected benefit—he believes that noni helped him bounce back from the flu much more quickly.

Dr. Robert Meery, a podiatrist in Williamstown, New Jersey has benefited greatly from noni. He says, "My specialty is medicine and surgery of the foot and ankle. I have been practicing in the Philadelphia–South New Jersey area for about eight years and I deal with many patients every day who suffer from chronic pain—whether it is due to arthritis, diabetes or other debilitating conditions. With most of these patients I must be careful with prescribing medications for pain relief due to interactions from other drugs they may be taking for other conditions, and/or their inability to ingest a prescribed anti-inflammatory due to gastrointestinal sensitivity. So noni has become a welcome alternative to prescription medications in my practice. What appeals to me most about noni is that it is without toxicity. I can offer it to my patients, loved ones, and friends without reservation."

Dr. Meery insisted on sharing another example of noni's effectiveness. "About a week and a half ago I noticed my secretary was having difficulty sitting and performing her office duties. She had been to an orthopedic surgeon several times due to lower back problems. She had also received several injections by an anesthesiologist in the spinal region. I offered her noni and within two hours, 75 percent of her pain was relieved. My patients have also noticed my excitement and enthusiasm when relating the benefits of noni and have accepted it overwhelmingly. In addition to my patients and loved ones, I have several colleagues in the medical field, ranging from general practitioners and chiropractors to orthopedic surgeons, who have accepted noni."

Dr. Meery can vouch for noni not only because he has seen it work for his patients, friends and colleagues—he has used the supplement himself! He explains, "Off and on over the past several years I have been suffering from degenerative joint disease in my neck area. I have also developed seasonal allergies. For approximately three weeks, I have been taking noni as-needed for these symptoms. Each time I take noni my symptoms are almost immediately relieved."

The quick symptomatic response seen by many noni users was also substantiated by two different Florida chiropractors, Dr. Alan Newman of the University Chiropractic Center, and Dr. Richard Smith.

FIBROMYALGIA

Margaret tells of her experience with noni. "Over the past ten years I have been suffering from an illness called fibromyalgia. This illness gives me daily muscle pain. I get inflammation in my arms, neck, and chest. It also makes me very tired. I've tried everything in the past, from Advil to steroids. Then recently, a friend of mine, Cathy, introduced me to noni, and I started taking it about 4 weeks ago. In the past, I found that most natural remedies take several months before you see any results, and usually the results are pretty minimal. But noni took only a few days. I noticed my energy start to increase and it lessened some of my food cravings. In the last week or so I have also noticed that my allergies to pollen and dust have decreased greatly. I guess you could say my results from noni have been great."

ARTHRITIS

Abigail, an 81-year-old client, went to Dr. Schechter with pains in her right shoulder and hip from arthritis and intermittent claudication (severe pain in calf muscles occurring during walking). These problems were especially distressing because she had enjoyed an active tennis game until the pain started. Due to indigestion and eating less, she became thin and frail. After taking noni for four weeks, she was walking smoothly and effortlessly up gentle hills, and the pains in her shoulder and hip were gone. She recently invited Dr. Schechter for an easy game of tennis. Neither party will inform me who the victor was.

Dale, of Boca Raton, Florida, says, "For the last five years I have been experiencing the onset of arthritis. Two years ago it became so severe in my thumbs and forefingers that I could no longer open a door without a lot of pain. I talked to my doctor about it and his advice was to take Motrin or endure the pain. My sister introduced me to noni about two weeks ago. I began taking it a week ago and within 36 hours, I regained full motion of my thumbs and fingers and the pain is gone—thanks to noni and the people who told us about it." Like Dale, 80 percent of the more than 8,000 patients in our survey reported that they experienced arthritic relief when taking noni.

Dale's wife, Diane, says, "Ten years ago I was diagnosed with gouty arthritis in my feet and hips and it was very painful, to say the least. When my husband and I started on noni, I was very skeptical, but I tried it anyway. Within the first 24 hours the pain lessened so much I could hardly believe it. Within 36 hours the pain was totally gone. I can get up in the morning and walk around without hobbling for up to an hour sometimes. Noni is wonderful! I wish it had been around years ago."

INFLAMMATION

Lisa, of Redding, California, says, "I would like to thank my friends for introducing me to noni. When they first had me try it for my knee, I was skeptical because I had been told surgery was the only answer. I have to admit, though, that after taking noni, the inflammation in my knee decreased and I have much more freedom of movement."

Even better, however, are results of noni on Lisa's neck. She explains, "I have had two surgeries on my neck. The first was a cervical fusion due to a herniated disc that I sustained in an autompbile accident. I also suffered major damage to the muscles in my neck and back in the accident. The second was a cervical laminectomy on a second herniated disc that had been weakened by the first injury. I now have aggravated my arthritis as a result of the injuries and subsequent surgeries. Neck pain has been an everyday constant in my life for the past seven years and, according to the doctor, unavoidable without strong medication that could ultimately damage my kidneys and liver. I chose to endure the pain rather than cause irreversible damage to my organs. While taking noni to help my knee, I realized that the stiffness and pain in my neck was greatly reduced and, on some days, completely gone. I cannot tell you what a welcome surprise this has been. I get the benefits of prescription drugs without the dangers."

WEIGHT LIFTING AND ASSOCIATED MUSCLE ACHES

Jack, from Portland, Oregon, states, "As an athlete and weight lifter, I know how it feels when your muscles ache. The other day I did a heavy leg workout, and for two days my legs hurt. Then I took noni for a couple of days and, let me tell you, the muscle aches were completely gone."

Terry, an acquaintance of Jack's, says, "I have had knee problems from squatting heavy weight during my workout. I started taking noni and noticed my pain was reduced by about 70 percent."

CARPAL TUNNEL SYNDROME

Cindy, a registered nurse from Minneapolis, has experienced various benefits from noni. The first was relief of carpal tunnel syndrome. She says, "A couple of months ago I was experiencing some pain down my left arm and my left hand. I was also experiencing some numbness and tingling while I was asleep at night. I went to the chiropractor and he diagnosed me with carpal tunnel syndrome. He suggested I take some extra vitamin B6 and wear a wrist immobilizer splint on my left arm at night while I slept. It did help at times, but it got old. My husband was taking noni for a little while and suggested I take it and see what it would do for me. I was also experiencing some neck and shoulder pain as well. I took noni for about four days and one morning—I couldn't believe it—I woke up and told my husband that my left arm didn't hurt as much as it had. This was exciting because I don't have to sleep with that splint on my wrist. The pain is down and it feels pretty good—and I am thrilled with that."

PMS

Cindy also explains how noni helped relieve her PMS symptoms. "About a week ago I started my period and like many other women throughout the United States I suffer from PMS where you have the mood swings and depression. I was having severe cramping and I would take pain pills and sometimes they would have to have a little codeine with them. While I was on vacation I started my period and started having cramps and I decided to try noni and within a half hour my cramps were gone and I felt great. I have been really pleased with noni and all the benefits it has given me."

FATIGUE, ENERGY AND INCREASED FEELING OF WELL-BEING

Ron, an investment banker from Sacramento, California, says, "Every morning I start my day with food supplements. The combination gives me an energy lift that is absolutely second to none. I have also found that I don't have the ups and downs that coffee and other products with a lot of caffeine give me. The energy lasts throughout the day and gives me the ability to put much more effort into my everyday activities. I have been able to work out much more intensely for longer periods of time. Recently I added noni and it has helped my post-workout recovery time dramatically. I am definitely not as sore after strenuous workouts. The overall natural lift I have from taking noni has enabled me to get much more accomplished, and the significantly reduced fatigue is unbelievable. I can't wait to tell everyone I know about this incredible supplement."

Similar to Ron, 79 percent of the more than 8,000 noni users surveyed reported an increased feeling of well-being after taking noni. And an incredible 91 percent reported an increased energy level after taking noni.

Dr. Schechter's case studies are just a small sampling of the good things noni has done for people with chronic or debilitating conditions. Again and again, people scratch their heads in disbelief at the wonderful effects that noni has on their ailments; most have become believers of noni, and many call it the miracle medicine fruit.

6

Noni's Mechanism of Action: Basic Research

While the precise mechanisms by which noni works are not fully understood, noni does contain a number of substances—enzymes (like proxeroninase), building blocks (like proxeronine), and as a small amount of the alkaloid xeronine—that are believed to play a pivotal role in good health. Scientists speculate that there may be a number of different agents in noni that act in a synergistic manner to produce desirable effects. Research indicates that one way noni exerts its healing action is as an adaptogen. That is, noni goes to the places in the body where cells function abnormally and helps them to function more normally. Research also indicates strengthen the immune system, regulating cell function and cellular regeneration of damaged cells. Since noni seems to operate on the very basic and critical cellular level, it may be useful for a wide variety of conditions. I have learned many things about noni from Dr. Schechter and from the stories of his patients:

- Noni stimulates the production of T-cells in the immune system, which play a pivotal role in fighting off disease.
- Noni acts to enhance immune system function, involving macrophages and lymphocytes—vital parts of the body's natural defenses.
- Noni has been shown to be effective against many types of bacteria.
- Noni has unique anti-pain effects.
- Noni inhibits precancer function and appears to inhibit the growth of tumors in animal models. It appears to allow abnormal cells to function more normally.

In addition to Dr. Schechter's findings, I also believe that one mechanism through which noni exerts its healing action is through normalizing abnormal energy levels. The rest of this book examines the ways that noni and its principal constituents function to help the body heal itself and fight disease. Thus are the secrets of noni unlocked.

THE XERONINE-PROXERONINE CONNECTION

Noni has generated much interest among nutritionists, doctors, and other health professionals because of some of its key components. The main ingredient found in noni is proxeronine, which, along with proxeroninase and serotonin, is converted to xeronine. Xeronine is a pivotal ingredient in a wide range of normal biochemical reactions that helps the body heal itself. Xeronine, which is also found in small amounts in noni, helps damaged and sick cells normalize their function, thereby facilitating their repair.

Until the 1950s, there was little information on either noni or its valuable components. Dr. Ralph Heinicke did extensive research, first at the Pineapple Research Institute, and then at the Dole Company in Hawaii and for several dozen pharmaceutical companies interested in these products. For the first time, he is now releasing a portion of his unpublished data and observations.

FIRST THERE WAS BROMELAIN

When you consider the extremely complex nature of the biochemical reactions involved in the biosynthesis of the alkaloid xeronine, it seems understandable why this system has escaped attention for so long. While at the Pineapple Research Institute, Dr. Heinicke researched and isolated a substance contained in pineapple which resulted in the patent and production of commercial bromelain. Initially, he studied only its protease (protein enzyme) activity. However, he soon received reports from other researchers about certain unusual and highly desirable medicinal properties of bromelain that are not present in other commercial protease preparations. He concluded from these reports that bromelain must contain some additional unknown active ingredients.

It took Dr. Heinicke many years to discover the nature of the unknown ingredients, but he and his research team finally found why commercial bromelain works. It is successful not because of its protease activity, but because of a phytonutrient called proxeronine, which the body converts to xeronine. Although pineapple plants in Hawaii contain some proxeronine, the richest source comes from noni. Noni juice has 800 times more proxeronine than its nearest competitor, which is ripe virgin pineapple.

Noni was one of the plants which Dr. Heinicke investigated in 1957 as a possible competitor of bromelain. In the 1980s, noni fruit was determined to be the best and richest source of the principal active ingredients in the xeronine system. I spent about a year doing a worldwide search for scientific research, other data, and case studies to see if and how noni worked as a therapeutic agent. Doctors reported that noni helped many people with cancer, heart disease, stroke, diabetes, weakened immune system, digestive problems, energy problems, weight problems, burns, addictions, hair and skin problems, and others. As I was collecting data—particularly case studies—one of the questions that haunted me was how noni could possibly help all these people with so many diverse health problems. I concluded that it does not help everyone, and it does not help with all of these health problems. But 78 percent of the over 8,000 noni users reported that it helped them in some way; in fact, it helped them so much that 69 percent said that they would not give up their noni. In earlier parts of the book, we discussed the conditions against which noni has been shown to effective (see Table 3). Now we will discuss some of the basic research that lead to noni's use in fighting these conditions

EARLY BROMELAIN RESEARCH

Many people think that data from pharmaceutical manufacturers are more reliable than anecdotal reports. Several major drug companies in the United States, Germany, and Switzerland found commercial bromelain to be highly effective and safe in treating a wide range of ailments—the same ailments that noni helps. Their findings indicate that an important ingredient is present in certain plant products. In other words, the pharmaceutical houses proved that a food supplement could help many ailments, even though they did not know the chemical nature of the specific ingredient or how it operates in the body.

Dr. Heinicke reports that the director of one of the major United States drug companies stated in 1957 that the discovery of the value of bromelain ranked among the major pharmaceutical discoveries of the last 50 years. Dr. Heinicke's first major drug customer planned to use a solution of bromelain as a rapidly acting agent that provided relief for severe menstrual cramps in less than 30 seconds. The director of this company was so impressed with bromelain's effectiveness for this condition that he approved further research into the action of bromelain on a wide variety of other medical problems. (Unfortunately, today's commercial bromelain contains only about 3 percent of the active material—proxeronine—that made bromelain so pharmacologically active at that time.)

In further testing, the company found that the irrigation of large cancerous tumors with bromelain solution caused a rapid regression of the tumor. Another benefit was demonstrated by a boy who was seriously ill with emphysema. When treated with bromelain mist, he recovered quickly. Scientists found that combining bromelain with antibiotics enabled them to achieve better results with lower doses of the drugs. The same results have now been reported with noni. In fact, the survey of over 8,000 noni users showed that after taking noni, 78 percent reported an improvement of their respiratory problems.

Dr. Heinicke speculates that the pharmaceutical company's failure to pursue the project was due largely to not knowing how long it would take or how expensive it would be to determine the actual pharmacological agent that made commercial bromelain so valuable. The story is an interesting example of the complicated and unpredictable nature of research dealing with natural products.

For the final double-blind test required for FDA approval of the proposed drug, the drug company asked Dr. Heinicke to purify commercial bromelain. Three months later, when the results of the very extensive double blind tests were evaluated, they found that the purified bromelain had little or no effect on healing. Apparently, the protein purification process removed the ingredient responsible for the dramatic pharmacological activity of the original commercial bromelain. We now know that the nutraceutical removed was proxeronine, the same substance abundantly found in noni, and the apparent reason for noni's impressive therapeutic capabilities.

Although the drug company wanted to establish a large cooperative research project with Dole to discover the nature of the material that the purification process had removed, Dole had other plans. A different drug company already had received FDA approval for selling an enteric-coated bromelain tablet for the control of inflammation. Dr. Heinicke said that Dole preferred to continue receiving its current profits rather than gamble on a larger income after expending additional unknown research expenses.

During the next ten years, Dr. Heinicke, who has no training in commercial pharmacology, worked closely with Gus Martin, the research director of the drug company that was selling enteric-coated bromelain to treat inflammation. Although Gus Martin's theory about the physiological action of bromelain was incorrect, he was a vigorous and imaginative research director whose laboratory produced an immense amount of valuable data that are still pertinent today. But he was not the only researcher working on bromelain.

NEW TECHNIQUE FOR TREATING BURN PATIENTS

Gerald Klein, M.D., a surgeon with Rommel's Panzer Corp in Africa during World War II, acquired extensive experience in treating severely burned patients in the

wake of fierce desert battles. During the African cam-
paign, he saw only patients who were dying, or wished
they could die, from their injuries. Dr. Klein vowed that
if he ever survived the war, he would devote the remainder of his life to finding a more humane way of treating
severely burned patients.

After the war, he moved to the United States and studied different treatments. His most successful method
involved applying a 50 percent paste of bromelain
directly to burned skin and then, two hours later, scrap-
ing off the paste along with the dead skin. He then
immediately grafted new skin onto the cleansed surface.
Dr. Heinicke worked closely with Dr. Klein in evaluating
several different preparations of pineapple stem colloids. Colloids were found in the original commercial
bromelain. As the first drug company had discovered,
both Dr. Klein and Dr. Heinicke learned that purified
bromelain was absolutely worthless for treating burns.

THE SEARCH FOR THE
XERONINE SYSTEM

The research on bromelain was much like the classic
example of five blind men attempting to describe the
nature of an elephant. Since each had only felt a part of
the animal—a trunk, a foot, or a tail—each had an incorrect understanding of the whole. In the case of bromelain, every unproductive lead addressed only one small
part of a very complex problem.

In his search for the physiologically active component
of bromelain, Dr. Heinicke at first suggested that sero-

tonin (a brain neurotransmitter) was the critical factor. This simplistic proposal was feasible since both pineapple and bromelain are rich in the alkaloid serotonin. Although he quickly dropped this suggestion, he still believed—which was probably correct—that serotonin had to play some critical role in the body's production of xeronine.

This is particularly interesting because *Morinda citrifolia* (noni) is one of the 80 species that belong to one of the most medicinally efficacious plant families, Rubiaceae. Noni has the greatest serotonin-binding capacity in the Rubiaceae plant family. I became particularly interested in serotonin receptors and binding during my training and teaching years at the Johns Hopkins Medical School and Hospital. I saw several patients who were significantly helped with depression and/or migraine headaches after taking serotonin analogue drugs. However, the side effects these patients experienced included nausea, diarrhea, dizziness, anxiety, allergic reactions, and even arrhythmias (irregular heart beats), and were often more devastating than the original condition.

Today, many scientists believe that serotonin is indeed one component used in the biosynthesis of the alkaloid called xeronine. Although very good research on serotonin has been done at the biomedical science department of the University of Hawaii and elsewhere, the specific pathway for exactly how serotonin works in the human body is still not completely known.

I often wondered why a person experiences undesirable side effects from purified medication, but rarely suffers from side effects to natural food supplements. There is an interesting answer. The World Health Organization found that 25 percent of all major medicines used today are derived from natural sources: herbs, plants, fruits, and/or trees. There are 120 of these plant-based medications in use today. Ninety medications (75 percent) used in modern medicine today are exactly like the original plant medicine. And it is known that the closer the modern medicine resembles the plant medicine, the fewer the side effects. This is true for noni, which has over 140 different ingredients. Mother Nature is by far the most effective and efficient pharmacist and medicine-maker in the world. God's design is truly godly.

I still have not told you why I believe noni can work so well, and without any significant side effects. It is, I believe, because Mother Nature put together in herbs, plants, fruit, etc., the perfect natural balance. One ingredient balances another in precise amounts and spatial and energy relationships. I believe that the more than 140 ingredients in noni act synergistically as accessory activating factors that bind to different receptors, all of which work in unison to prevent side effects.

Before I retired from practicing medicine for 30 years and being involved with over 30,000 patient-visits, I used natural food supplements instead of synthetic medication whenever I could. I believe that natural is better than unnatural. But if what we're finding out about noni and other natural food supplements is true, why did the pharmaceutical corporations isolate what they mistakenly thought was the active ingredient in bromelain (protease) instead of using a food supplement from noni fruit or even pineapple? Here is one possible explanation that people have told me. Pharmaceutical companies cannot patent fruits, herbs, plants, trees or other God-given nutrients. No patent means no big profits protected by government agencies. No multi-million dollar executive bonuses. No large contributions to politicians. Because of this, such companies would lose their special-interest status, and fair competition from supplemental and alternative medicine would flourish. This could lead to people taking more food supplements as preventive medicine with less illness, less patent medication sold, and less pharmaceutical profits.

Since Dr. Heinicke knew that purifying bromelain by certain techniques removed the active factor, he reasoned that the critical ingredient had to be lipophilic, or readily dissolvable in fat solvents. Later, he gave this crystalline material the name *proxeronine.* The richest source of this compound is the noni fruit.

Dr. Heinicke now estimates the amount of proxeronine which he obtained from pineapple samples in 1953 was greater than the total amount of other proteins present. (In fact, he later determined that noni has 800 times more proxeronine than pineapple). At that time, he was not interested in proxeronine and considered it an inconvenient contaminant in his efforts to isolate pure protein enzymes. Incidentally, Dr. Heinicke mentioned that these early samples of bromelain that were originally distributed to drug companies showed a physiological activity that has never been equaled by any commercial bromelain produced from 1957 to the present. That is because the bromelain at that time contained proxeronine.

The large size of the proxeronine (molecule molecular weight greater than 17,000) was the major problem that prevented the determination of its chemical structure. When Dr. Heinicke again isolated this molecule in 1974, he sent samples of the crystals to a laboratory specializing in the identification of organic molecules. The laboratory reported that the molecule was like no other molecule it had worked with or knew about, and that to finish the analysis it would require a large research grant. Today, with new equipment and techniques, a well-equipped laboratory could probably work out the chemical structure within a few months.

ISOLATING PURE XERONINE

Dr. Heinicke first isolated pure xeronine in 1977 while working at Jintan-Dolph, Japan. During the purification of different fractions isolated from commercial bromelain, he found one fraction that showed excellent biological activity. After additional purification, he finally had a flask that looked empty but had a strong nicotine-like odor. His colleague took the seemingly empty flask and subjected it to the same tests that he had developed for measuring the physiological activity of commercial bromelain. He reported that the solution with the odor was as physiologically active as the rest of the previous active fractions. From all indications, this was the long-sought-for physiologically active factor in bromelain, as well as in many other pharmacologically active plant extracts. I suspect that what was present was concentrated proxeronine mixed with a minute amount of xeronine.

Nevertheless, the scientific community requires more than odor as evidence of a discovery. Even though Dr. Heinicke had a commitment to return to Hawaii to work on a Hawaii state grant aimed at finding new opportunities to increase the profitability of pineapple fields, he stayed several extra weeks in Japan in an attempt to finish the project. Unfortunately, though the research was progressing rapidly, time and money ran out.

Consequently, Dr. Heinicke returned to Hawaii, where he had the luxury of working with a different order of raw material to isolate the active component. Instead of working with pounds of protein enzymes as his starting material, he had access from Dole to about 25 tons of pineapple stems. These studies eventually led to the isolation of about 50 mg of pure crystalline xeronine. These crystals were initially beautiful transparent crystals. After a day, the crystals turned to a silver color. These were even more attractive than the original crystals. The next day, they turned black. A pure solution of xeronine crystals showed an even more rapid disintegration than the crystals themselves. Initially, the solution was absolutely colorless. Within four hours, the solution became pink and then red. By the next day, the solution was black and all physiological activity has disappeared. (If noni juice turns dark black from its natural brown color, then the noni has lost its biological activity and is essentially useless.)

Since Dr. Heinicke knew that the crystals and solutions of the crystals were unstable and since he knew that making the crystals posed no problem, he decided to first prove that pure xeronine was the actual physiologically active ingredient in the body, even though proxeronine was the primary and most abundant ingredient in the noni extract. For his definitive test, he chose to use the foreign alkaloid tetrodotoxin, a highly poisonous substance found in the puffer fish.

Tetrodotoxin is in fact a potent poison, a fact fully documented by chemists. It acts as a powerful nerve toxin in killing mice. The death throes involve a frenzied, uncoordinated spasm of activity that generally ends with a final leap into the air followed by death. Previously, there was no known antagonist for this type of poisoning. Toxicologists long maintained that all of the supertoxins must be analogous to a normal body regulator, which they then poison.

On the basis of this belief, Heinicke hypothesized that tetrodotoxin must have a size and shape similar to the body's own alkaloids. His theory was that it blocks the body's own alkaloids from activating the receptor sites. If this hypothesis were correct, a combination of tetrodotoxin and xeronine should be nontoxic.

The results were dramatic, conclusive, and in one respect, surprising. As he had anticipated, Dr. Heinicke found that 100 percent of the mice that had been given only tetrodotoxin died in less than a minute in the typical nerve-poisoning death throes. In contrast, 100 percent of the mice given the mixture of tetrodotoxin and xeronine survived. What was completely unexpected and surprising was how they survived.

Mice given an intraperitoneal injection (an injection in the abdominal cavity) of even a harmless saline solution act as if they feel uncomfortable. When a mouse is returned to its cage after being injected, it immediately burrows into the shavings to wait until the discomfort of the injection wears off. By contrast, all of the mice given xeronine (this included both the group of mice given the mixture of tetrodotoxin and xeronine as well as the group of mice give only xeronine) remained very active when they returned to their cages. This behavior was so striking that a visitor from another laboratory who happened to see these mice shortly after they were injected with xeronine asked Dr. Heinicke where he obtained such intelligent mice!

Dr. Heinicke recalls that she still had remaining a few milliliters of the xeronine solution after the experiment. Since he knew it was harmless would be worthless the next day when it turned black, he decided he had nothing to lose and drank it. He noticed nothing particularly different. But, that evening he started reading chemical abstracts, a chore that generally was so tedious that he could rarely cover more than a few pages at a time. After he had been reading for some time, he glanced at his watch. It was three o'clock in the morning and he had gone through several back issues. Just as Dr. Heinicke found, the results of our survey of over 8,000 noni users showed similar results. In fact, 73 percent reported significantly more energy, greater alertness, and more clarity than before they had used noni.

Within about a week, Dr. Heinicke had examined the action of pure crystalline xeronine in almost all of the standard and laboratory tests that research workers had been using to evaluate the effectiveness of bromelain. These included the effects on bleeding time, on dye diffusion, on aggregation of blood platelets exposed to adenosinediphosphate (ADP), and on milk clotting action. He found the test results from bromelain and xeronine to be identical.

One critical part of the xeronine system still remains to be covered, namely the enzyme proxeroninase, which performs one of the last steps in the biosynthesis of xeronine. Proxeroninase is a member of a rather ubiquitous class of enzymes, the lysozymes.

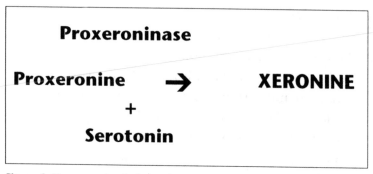

Figure 1: How xeronine is formed

PROXERONINASE AND PROXERONINE

In 1954, Dr. Heinicke unknowingly isolated from the pineapple fruit an enzyme that would later be named proxeroninase. As mentioned previously, proxeroninase is the enzyme necessary to complete the process by which xeronine is produced. Figure 1 demonstrates how proxeroninase combines with proxeronine and serotonin to form xeronine, the active compound in noni that helps abnormally functioning cells function more normally.

POSTULATED ACTION OF XERONINE

Dr. Heinicke told me of a study done by an excellent gynecologist, the late Dr. Gerard of France. Because of his interest in cancer research, and because one of his patients absolutely refused to have a mastectomy for an advanced case of breast cancer, Dr. Gerard decided to conduct a clinical trial involving this woman. He asked whether she would be willing to try an alternate treatment. His theory was that if a person took three pills of enteric-coated bromelain at intervals of every two hours while awake, something in bromelain would enter the bloodstream and make cancer cells behave similarly to normal cells.

The patient was skeptical but felt that she had nothing to lose, especially when Dr. Gerard assured her there were no adverse side effects to the pills. She agreed to begin treatment.

Initially, her improvement was dramatic. Photograms taken every week for one month after the start of the treatment showed a steady decrease in the size of the cancerous breast ulcer. If the same treatment had been continued at this point, Dr. Gerard estimated that the ulcer should have disappeared within another month.

The woman told Dr. Gerard that with this massive dose of pills, she had observed in her stool that some of them were going unabsorbed through her intestinal tract. So he made a change in the method of administering the drug. To avoid this waste of pills, he modified his prescription for her. He ground a batch of pills in a mortar, placed a two-hour dose in a gelatin capsule, and told her to take the new capsules every two hours.

The following week's photogram showed that the ulcer had begun growing vigorously again. In fact, it was growing faster than it had been decreasing in size during the initial weeks of treatment. Dr. Gerard immediately put the patient back on the same high dose of enteric-coated pills, which was three pills every two hours. The following week, the photograms showed that her ulcer was again decreasing in size. After two months of treatment, all visible signs of cancer had disappeared.

Dr. Gerard told her that even though the cancerous breast lesion had disappeared, she should continue to take bromelain for at least two more years. His theory was that some part of bromelain temporarily causes cancer cells to behave as normal cells as long as this component remains present in the blood stream. He theorized that a substance in the enteric-coated bromelain released something in the intestinal tract that was absorbed and transferred through the vein to the liver. This material then circulated through the blood stream and did something that made breast cancer cells behave similarly to normal cells. In other words, they did not continue dividing longer than they should. He believed that a permanent remission would require sufficient time for the body to replace all of the cancer cells with normally acting cells.

Destroying the integrity of the enteric coating of the pills through the grinding process completely destroyed the biological action of bromelain for this medical problem. Dr. Heinicke reasoned that either one or both of two things happened. Either 1) a critical enzyme (proxeroninase) contained in the bromelain capsule was destroyed in the stomach; or 2) a critical component in bromelain, namely proxeronine, was released and absorbed as a single massive active dose in the enteric coated pills, instead of being absorbed slowly over a two-hour period, as it would have been with the crushed pills. The slow, continuous absorption of proxeronine was not effective, whereas the high pulsatile dose was very effective. The rapid diminution of the size of the breast cancer when the patient began taking the enteric-coated pills again suggests that the proper treatment was effective and that this was not a spontaneous cure. This single case, however dramatic, should not be considered the sole treatment for breast cancer or any other cancer.

Dr. Heinicke believes that noni helps the normalization of abnormal functioning cells by delivering to the body the necessary ingredients, which the body then puts together to make xeronine. Xeronine exhibits positive effects on cells that result in most people feeling better. Understanding how the body makes xeronine through the process of biosynthesis is essential to understanding how noni works.

The major building blocks involved in our body's biosynthesis of xeronine are proxeronine, proxeroninase—an enzyme needed in the biosynthesis of xeronine—and serotonin. Your body contains all of them, but proxeronine is in short supply. Here is how Dr. Heinicke believes the biosynthesis of xeronine works.

Under usual circumstances, the liver stores proxeronine. About every two hours, the brain sends a signal to the liver to release a large "slug" of proxeronine. The various body organs then absorb from the bloodstream

Toning down over-secreting mucus membranes
Representative Examples:
Sinusitis, asthma, bronchitis and chronic post-nasal drip.

Toning down increased production of stomach acids
Representative Examples:
Gastric and duodenal ulcers, gastritis, and esophageal reflux of gastric acid.

Autoimmune disease
Representative Examples:
Rheumatoid arthritis, psoriasis, diabetes mellitus Type 2, thyroiditis, Crohn's disease and lupus erythematosus.

Infections
Representative Examples:
Herpes types 1 & 2, chronic hepatitis, pelvic inflammatory disease, postviral syndrome, pancreatitis, viral thyroiditis, and yeast, mold and fungus infections such as athlete's foot, yeast vaginitis, thrush, and many other mycotic (fungus) infections.

Progressive disorganization of specific tissues
Representative Examples:
Uterine fibroids, atherosclerosis, diverticular disease, warts, and the breakdown of surveillance against malignant cells, which can lead to cancer.

Immunodeficiency
Representative Examples:
Viral diseases like HIV and Epstein-Barr, and chronic candidiasis, lack of vital energy and AES, which is an altered energy response to handling of stress and which comes from my work at the Johns Hopkins Medical Institutions.

Altered energy state
Representative Examples:
Lack of vital energy and AES, which is an altered energy response to handling stress and which comes from my work with patients at the Johns Hopkins Medical Institutions.

Table 5. Clinical conditions for which noni can be used

an amount of proxeronine sufficient to produce the amount of xeronine they require for the repairing process. Normally, cells contain sufficient amounts of the other biochemicals required for the synthesis of xeronine—generally, only proxeronine is in short supply.

All is fine unless there is an increased requirement for xeronine in a tissue or organ. Any major stress could cause this. Precancerous abnormal cell activity or any number of health problems, including physical and/or

---

Digestive system
Representative Examples:
Diarrhea, worms, nausea and food poisoning.

Respiratory system
Representative Examples:
Cough, sore throat, tuberculosis, cholera and infant chest colds.

Inflammation
Representative Examples:
Arthritis, tendonitis, and fibromyalgia.

Cardiovascular system
Representative Examples:
Hypertension, heart muscle thickening (such as left ventricular hypertrophy).

Analgesic
Representative Examples:
Most types of pain.

Skin/Hair conditions
Representative Examples:
Burns, wounds, ulcers, abscesses, cellulitis, swelling, ring worm, boils, sores, scalp conditions including dandruff, and itching.

Febrile conditions
Representative Examples:
Most of the febrile conditions regardless of cause.

Other conditions
Representative Examples:
Tumors, broken bones, liver disease, asthma, dysentery, and sick cells with too much acid.

Table 6. Body systems that were reported to have responded positively to noni treatment

emotional problems, or fungus infections and toxins, may bring about this need for more xeronine. When this occurs the demand for xeronine increases dramatically. The liver usually does not have enough extra stored proxeronine to send to damaged cells. The tissues of these cells have an abundant supply of proxeroninase and serotonin; what is lacking is proxeronine. Noni juice is helpful because it contains plenty of proxeronine.

I took the liberty to simplify a very complex system where many other biochemical, hormonal, and immunological reactions are simultaneously taking place. Dr. Heinicke gave us the biochemistry of the noni-xeronine connection. Dr. Gerson postulates that noni demonstrates its clinical capabilites through the noni-xeronine-proxeronine connection. Table 5 lists the specific conditions that have been reported to respond positively to treatment with noni. This was very often in connection with other traditional medical treatments.

As cited previously, Dr. Gerson completed clinical trials with noni on patients with high blood pressure and on others with high cholesterol. Noni had a positive effect on lowering blood pressure and cholesterol levels. This effect could only be enhanced by also following the tradtional diet, exercise, and medical guidelines. He knew that other patients had used it successfully for menstrual cramps, gastric ulcers, and diabetes. Since he found that noni had the best medicinal results of the entire Rubiaceae family, he documented how Rubiacea aided other body systems, generally functioning to enhance the activity of other medical compounds. They include the following.

ACTIONS OF FREE XERONINE AND PROXERONINE ON THE STOMACH MUSCLES

It is said that noni strengthens and normalizes weak stomach muscles. In 1925, Dr. Howard W. Haggard of Yale University showed that of all the fruit products that he tested, canned pineapple juice was the only one that contained a substance that increased and strengthened the motility, or movement, of weak stomach muscles. Since there is no protease (a group of proteolytic enzymes that aid in the breakdown of proteins) in pineapple juice, it couldn't possibly be associated with this action, as previously thought.

In 1973, by which time Dr. Heinicke had developed an early version of the xeronine system concept, he compared the activity of xeronine and proxeronine on gastric motility. For this experiment, he placed a strip of stomach muscle from a mouse in a tensiometer, a device to measure muscle tension. He could add samples that he wanted tested to the constant flowing stream of saline (salt water) and nutrients.

The results were striking. As soon as the stream of solution containing the xeronine reached the muscle, both the frequency, or rate, and the amplitude, or strength, of the muscular contractions increased. As soon as he switched to the standard saline solution, the frequency and amplitude of contractions immediately returned to baseline. By contrast, as soon as the stream of solution containing the proxeronine reached the muscle, nothing happened. Then about two seconds later, both the frequency and the amplitude of the contractions increased to the same extent as had occurred with the xeronine solution. When he switched back to the saline solution, both the frequency and amplitude of the contractions continued for two seconds before returning to baseline. He repeated this experiment many times with identical results.

(ethylthomethyl) benzene
1-butanol
1-hexanol
1-methoxy-2-formyl-3-hydroxyan-
thraquinone
2,5-undecadien-1-ol
2-heptanone
2-methyl-2-butenyl decanoate
2-methyl-2-butenyl hexanoate
2-methyl-3,5,6-trihydroxyan-
thraquinone-6-ß-primeveroside
2-methyl-3,5,6-trihydroxyan-
thraquinones
2-methylbutanoic acid
2-methylpropanoic acid
24-methylcycloartanol
24-methylenecholesterol
24-methylenecycloartanyl linoleate
3-hydroxyl-2-butanone
3-hydroxymorindone
3-hydroxymorindone-6-ß-primevero-
side
3-methyl-2-buten-1-ol
3-methyl-3-buten-1-ol
3-methylthiopropanoic acid
5,6-dihydroxylucidin
5,6-dihydroxylucidin-3- ß-primeveroside
5,7-acacetin7-O-ß-D-(+)-glucopyra-
noside
5,7-dimethylapigenin-4'-O-ß-D-
D(+)=galactopyranoside
6,8-dimethoxy-3-methyl
anthraquinone-1,-O-ß-rhamnosyl
glucopyranoside
6-dodeceno-y-lactone
7-hydroxy-8-methoxy-2-methylan-
thraquinone
8,11,14-eicosatrienoic acid
acetic acid
alizarin
alkaloids
anthragallol 1,2-dimethyl ether
anthraquinones
antrhagallol 2,3-dimethyl ehter
asperuloside
benzoic acid
benzyl alcohol
butanoic acid
calcium

campesteryl glycoside
campesteryl linoleyl glycoside
campesteryl palmitate
campesteryl palmityl glycoside
campestrol
carbonate
carotene
cycloartenol
cycloartenol linoleate
cycloartenol palmitate
damnacanthal
decanoic acid
elaidic acid
ethyl decanoate
ethyl hexanoate
ethyl octanoate
ethyl palmitate
eugenol
ferric iron
gampesteryl linoleate
glucose
glycosides
heptanoic acid
hexadecane
hexanamide
hexanedioic acid
hexanoic acid
hexose
hexyl hexanoate
iron
isobutyric acid
isocaproic acid
isofucosterol
isofucosteryl linoleate
isolaveric acide
lauric acid
limonene
linoleic acid
lucidin
lucidin-3- ß-primeveroside
magnesium
methyl 3-methylthio-propanoate
methyl decanoate
methyl elaidate
methyl hexanoate
methyl octanoate
methyl oleate
methyl palmitate
morenone-1
morenone-2

Table 7: Nutraceuticals identified in noni (cont. on next page)

morindadiol	ricinoleic acid
morindanigrine	rubiadin
morindin	rubiadin-1-methyl ether
morindone	scopoletin
morindone-6-ß-primeveroside	sitosterol
mucilaginous matter	sitosteryl glycoside
myristic acid	sitosteryl linoleate
n-butyric acid	sitosteryl linoleyl glycoside
n-valeric acid	sitosteryl palmitate
nonanoic acid	sitosteryl palmityl glycoside
nordamnacanthal	sodium
octadecenoic acid	sorandjidiol
octanoic acid	ß-sitosterol
oleic acid	stearic acid
palmitic acid	sterols
paraffin	stigmasterol
pectins	stigmasteryl glycoside
pentose	stigmasteryl linoleate
phenolic body	stigmasteryl linoleyl glycoside
phosphate	stigmasteryl palmitate
physcion	stigmasteryl palmityl glycoside
physcion-8-O[{L-arabinopyranosyl} (1-	terpenoids
3) {ß-D- g-D- galactopyranosyl (1-6)	trioxymethylanthraquinone
{ß-D- galactopyranoside}]	undecanoic acid
potassium	ursolic acid
protein	vitamin C
resins	vomifoliol
rhamnose	wax

Table 7 (cont.): Nutraceuticals identified in noni
Source: Hirazumi, A., Ph.D. dissertation (see bibliography). Used by permission.

These data suggest that xeronine causes an immediate muscular response, whereas proxeronine first has to diffuse into the muscle strip and then be converted to xeronine before it has its positive effect.

All the components of the xeronine system are found in noni, and Dr. Heinicke believes that proxeronine from noni is the critical factor that helps the body to heal itself. It does so by supplying the body with ample amounts of proxeronine, which can then be synthesized to the alkaloid xeronine.

He further believes that this xeronine alkaloid fits onto a cell receptor site adjacent to the adsorption site for beta-endorphin. As a result, most people feel better. Our survey of over 8,000 noni users showed that after taking noni, 79 percent reported an increased sense of well-being. It is not surprising that people with health problems require more proxeronine and therefore take more noni.

Over 140 isolated nutraceuticals—products extracted from natural sources—that play a large integrative role in noni's effectiveness have now been identified in the different parts of noni. These are included in Table 7.

7

Clinical Uses
of Noni Juice

For use in the United States, the noni fruit is prepared as a food supplement, usually in juice form. Although the plant is very bitter and has a foul odor, the noni juice supplement is very palatable in taste and smell because of the addition of natural grape, blueberry, and other juices.

To maintain the integrity of noni's actions, the following natural constituents must be included in the noni supplement: naturally occurring vitamins, minerals, trace elements, beneficial alkaloids, plant sterols, enzymes, cofactors and phytonutrients. For best results, no additives, artificial ingredients, or preservatives should be added. (See Table 7 for a more complete list of noni nutraceuticals.) The richest noni grows in a tropical climate with direct sunlight. It grows best in rich volcanic soil that contains an abundance of calcium and selenium. In French Polynesia (Tahiti), noni grows very well in its native state.

SUGGESTED DOSAGES

Table 8 lists the recommended loading, maintenance, and/or preventive doses of noni juice to be taken for both adults and children. According to Dr. Heinicke, there need be no dose adjustment for weight because noni is stored in and released by the liver. Noni should be taken just before breakfast and just before dinner. Dr. Heinicke's results were obtained by using a combination of 89 percent pure juice from the noni plant, combined with 11 percent pure grape, blueberry, and other blended juices. This specific combination of juices allows for a pleasant taste and smell.

Before starting noni or any food supplement, you should always consult your physician and/or health professional. For optimal improvement, some people need more noni, some need less. Your body will tell you. If you feel that you are not getting optimal improvement, increase your daily intake by taking an additional one-half ounce noni juice, half an hour before lunch for 7 days. Increase the dose every 7 days by one half ounce until you obtain the desired results or until you double your original starting dose. In the rare exception when you have no improvement after being on the double dose for six months, noni probably will not help you. For economic reasons, you should stop taking the loading dose. You might still benefit from taking the maintenance dose, which is also the preventive dose.

Loading Dose: Month 1	
Ounces of Noni Juice	
Adult (over 16 years)	
Before Breakfast	2
Before Dinner	2
Child (under 16 years)	
Before Breakfast	1
Before Dinner	1
Take before breakfast and dinner	
Therapeutic Dose: Month 2 through Month 6	
Ounces of Noni Juice	
Adult (over 16 years)	
Before Breakfast	2
Before Dinner	1
Child (under 16 years)	
Before Breakfast	1
Before Dinner	1/2
Take before breakfast and dinner	
Maintenance and Prevention: Month 7 and After	
Ounces of Noni Juice	
Adult (over 16 years)	
Before Breakfast	1
Before Dinner	1
Child (under 16 yrs.)	
Before Breakfast	1
Take before breakfast and dinner	

Table 8: Suggested loading, therapeutic and maintenance dosages for noni. Dosages for animals is the same as for children.

Summary

As I MENTIONED IN THE PREFACE, I SPENT MOST OF 1997 and 1998 researching both the scientific evidence and anectdotal material involving the island fruit noni to see if and how it works as a medicinal agent. I discovered that noni is associated with folkloric accounts of miraculous healings of an extremely wide range of physical and mental ailments. In conjunction with my research, I interviewed more than 40 doctors and other health professionals who had compiled data that collectively represented over 8,000 of their patients who had used or were using noni.

The result of this survey are certainly impressive. The doctors and other health professionals interviewed believed that noni helped 78 percent of those who took it for one or more problems. And side effects were minimal. Less than 5 percent had a slight belching, loose stools, or were allergic to the noni fruit and developed a slight rash. The belching and loose stools disappeared with lower doses; the rash cleared within 72 hours after having stopped taking noni.

In addition, these doctors and health professionals

also noted that noni appears to be safe for pregnant and/ or nursing mothers. Checking with your health profession is still prudent.

The survey also indicates that noni can be taken with all medications. There were no reported negative interactions from any of the doctors. In fact, in some situations, noni actually allowed other medications to act more efficiently. You should tell your health professional that you are taking noni, as your physician might want to decrease the dose of other medication(s) he/she is prescribing.

In sharing their experiences with me, these doctors and health practitioners provided valuable information about the dosage range that most helped the majority of the 6,240 out of the 8,000 people who had a positive response to noni (see Table 8 for these dosages). Ingestion of the noni also helped about 90 percent of the animals with a wide range of health problems.

Other data gathered for the production of this book indicate that noni is a powerful nutraceutical. One of its key compounds, xeronine, was discovered by Dr. Ralph Heinicke, and serves as a critical modifier for one or more of the body proteins and enzymes. Dr. Heinicke refers to the system in which xeronine is biosynthesized as the xeronine system. He believes that all of the building blocks for the xeronine system are contained in noni. Healthy people generally have adequate amounts of all of this system's components with the exception of proxeronine, which is frequently present in marginal amounts. A lack of proxeronine in our bodies may lead to the breakdown of normal body functions and ultimately lead to the formation of a wide variety of disorders, including some types of cancer, and disorders of the immune, cardiovascular, mental, endocrine and digestive systems. Dr. Heinicke's discovery of xeronine and the xeronine system has important ramifications for future research and health-care practices.

In summary, all of this focus on noni has yielded what Polynesian kahunas have known for ages: noni is a remarkable fruit, and scientists are steadily putting a legitimate stamp of approval on the plant and its medicinal abilities. Slowly but surely, the noni plant is shedding its mystical aura and becoming a viable and effective method to ease the pain and suffering caused by dozens of the most common ailments.

This book, hopefully, has helped you form an appreciation of the tropical fruit noni. Noni can make a difference in your life.

Bibliography

Abbott, L.A., (1992) La'au Hawaii: Traditional Hawaiian Uses of Plants, Bishop Museum Press, Honolulu, Hawaii, 3: 97-199.

Abbott, I. and Shimazu, C., (1985) The Geographic Origin of the Plants Most Commonly Used for Medicine by Hawaiians, Journal of Ethnopharmacology, 14: 213-22.

Bushnell, O.A., Fukuda, M., Makinodan, T., (1950) The Antibacterial Properties of Some Planta Med, 36: 186-187.

Bushnell, O.A., Fukuda, M., Makinodan, T., (1950) The Antibacterial Properties of Some Plants Found in Hawaii, Pacific Science, 4: 167-183.

Cox, Paul Alan, Polynesian Herbal Medicine . In P.A.Coxeronine and S.A. Banack [eds.], Islands, Plants, and Polynesians, Portland: Dioscorides Press, 1991.

Ditmar, Alexander, (1993) Morinda Citrifolia L., Use in Indigenous Samoan Medicine. Journal of Herbs, Spices and Medical Plants, Vol 1(3), 1993.

Elliott, S. and Brimacombe, J., (1987) The Medicinal Plants of Cunnung Leuser National Park, Indonesia. *Journal of Ethnopharmacology*, 19: 285-317. Elsevier Scientific Publisher Ireland, Ltd.

Ganal, C. and Hokama, Y. The Effect of noni Fruit Extract (Morinda Citrifolia, Indian Mulberry) on Thymocytes of BALB/c Mouse (Meeting Abstract). Nutrition and Cancer, Vol. II. Dept. of Pathology, John A. Burns School of Medicine, University of Hawaii, 4999-5002.

Guest, P.L., (1938) Samoan Trees, Appendix E. Mimeogr. The Museum, Honolulu, Hawaii. Frm Uhe 1974.24.

Hawaii Medical Journal, (1966) Evaluation of the Effectiveness of Ancient Hawaiian Medicine.

Health News, Vol. 4, No. 2. Triple R Publishing, Inc.

Healthy Matters, Vol. 4, No. 2, 1-4. Ryder Thompson Enterprises. 13. Healthy Pet, Vol. 5, No. 1, 1-4. Ryder Thompson Enterprises.

Heinicke, Doctor R.M., The Pharmacologically Active Ingredient of Noni, Bulletin of the National Tropical Botanical Garden, 1985.

Heinicke, Doctor R. M., October-December, 1997, Personal Communication. Louisville, KY.

Hiramatsu, Tomonori; Imoto, Masaya; Koyano, Takashi; Umezawa, Kazuo.

Induction of Normal Phenotypes in Ras-Transformed Cells by Damnacanthal From *Morinda citrifolia*. Cancer Letters, Vol. 73 , 1993.

Hirazumi, A., (1992) Antitumor Activity of *Morinda citrifolia* on IP Implanted Lewis Lung Carcinoma in Mice. Proceedings Annual Meeting of The American Association for Cancer Research, 33: 515.

Hirazumi, A., Furusawa, E., Chou, S.C., Hokama, Y.; Anticancer Activity of *Morinda citrifolia* (noni) on Intraperitoneally Implanted Lewis Lung Carcinoma in Syngeneic Mice. Proc. West Pharmacological Society, 37, 1994.

Hulbert, Dr. Richard, Personal Communication, December, 1997. Boise, ID.

Krauss, B., (1993) Plants in Hawaiian Culture, University of Hawaii Press, Honolulu, Hawaii, 103: 252.

Levand, Oscar. Some Chemical Constituents of *Morinda citrifolia* in Unpublished Doctoral Dissertation from the University of Hawaii, 1963.

Levand, O. and Larson, H.O., Some Chemical Constituents of Morinda Citrifolia, Planta Med, Vol. 36, 1979.

McCuddin, Ch.R., (1974) Samoan Medicinal Plants and Their Usage. Department of Medical Services, Government of American Samoa, Pago American Samoan.

McPherson, C. and McPherson, L., (1990) Samoan Medical Belief and Practice. Auckland University Press, Auckland.

Moorthy, N.K., Reddy, G.S.. Antiseptic, Vol. 56, 1990.

Morton, Julia F., The Ocean-Going noni, or Indian Mulberry and Some of Its Colorful Relatives, Economic Botany, Vol. 43(3), 1992.

Neal, M., (1965) In Gardens of Hawaii. Bishop Museum Press, Honolulu, Hawaii, 804

Noni, Polynesia's Natural Pharmacy. (1997) Pride Publishing, Vineyard, VT.

Powell, T., (1868) On Various Samoan Plants and Their Vernacular Names. Br. Foreign J. Bot., 278-285, 342-347, 355-370.

Russia, K. and Sriivastava, S.K., (1987) Antimicrobial Activity of Some Indian Medicinal Plants. Indian Journal of Pharmacological Science, Jan-Feb: 57-58.

Schechter, Dr. Steven, Hawaii Miracle Fruit, noni Fruit Table, September, 1997.

Schechter, Dr. Steven, Noni Booklet, September 23, 1997. Encinitas, CA.

Schechter, Dr. Steven, Personal communication, November-December, 1997.

Sim, Helen. The Isolation and Characterization of a Fluorescent Compound From the Fruit of Morinda Citrifolia (noni): Studies on the 5-ht Receptor System. Unpublished Master's Thesis from the University of Hawaii at Monoa, 1993.

Singh, Y., Ikahihifo, T., Panuve, Slatter, C., (1984) Folk Medicine in Tonga. A Study on the use of Herbal Medicines for Obstetric and Gynecological Conditions and Disorders. Journal of Ethnopharmacology, 12: 305-325.

Solomon, N., and M. Lipton: *Sick & Tired of Being Sick & Tired.* New York, Wyndwood Press, April 1989.

Tabrah, F.L. and Eveleth, B.M., Evaluation of the Effectiveness of Ancient Hawaiian Medicine. Hawaiian Medical Journal, 25, 1966.

TenBruggencate, Jan; Native Plants Can Heal Your Wounds. Honolulu Star Bulletin & Advertiser, Honolulu, Hawaii, Feb. 9, 1992.

Whistler, A., M.D., Polynesian Herbal Medicine. National Tropical Garden, Lawai, Kauai, Hawaii, 173-174.

Whistler, W., (1992) Tongan Herbal Medicine. Isle Botanica, Honolulu, Hawaii, 89-90.

Whistler, W.A., (1985) Traditional and Herbal Medicine in the Cook Islands. Journal of Ethnopharmacology, 13: 239-280.

Younos, Chafique; Rolland, Alain; Fleurentin, Jacques; Lanhers, Marie-Claire; Misslin, Rene; Mortier, Francois. Analgesic and Behavioral Effects of Morinda Citrifolia. Planta Med Vol. 56, 1990.